COPING IN A CHANGING WORLD™

BODY PIERCING AND TATTOOING

THE HIDDEN DANGERS OF BODY ART

Sarah Sawyer

ROSEN PUBLISHING®
New York

Published in 2007 by The Rosen Publishing Group, Inc.
29 East 21st Street, New York, NY 10010

First Edition

Library of Congress Cataloging-in-Publication Data

Sawyer, Sarah.
Body piercing and tattooing: the hidden dangers of body art / Sarah Sawyer.—1st ed.
p. cm.—(Coping in a changing world)
Includes bibliographical references and index.
ISBN-13: 978-1-4042-0947-3
ISBN-10: 1-4042-0947-6 (library binding)
1. Body piercing—Health aspects. 2. Tattooing—Health aspects. I. Title.
GN419.25.S28 2007
391.6'5—dc22

2006024487

Manufactured in the United States of America

Contents

CHAPTER ONE

A History of Body Art

TATTOOING IS AN EXAMPLE OF HOW A SMALL, REMOTE SOCIETY HAD A TREMENDOUSLY SIGNIFICANT IMPACT ON EUROPEAN CULTURE.

Body modification in the form of tattooing and piercing is more popular in the United States than ever before, a trend that started spiking in the 1990s and has since grown steadily. In fact, according to a 2003 poll by Harrison Interactive, 16 percent of Americans, or roughly 48 million people, have at least one tattoo.[1] For proof, you need only open the pages of any fashion magazine to see the many people who express themselves with body art. Recent generations may have limited their modifications to a single piercing on each ear or a discreetly placed tattoo, but today's body art enthusiasts proudly boast their ink and titanium in many new ways and in surprising new places.

For the last thirty years, body modifications have been inching their way into mainstream society. Among the variety of people who today proudly sport tattoos include former secretary of state George P. Schultz, writer John Irving, actor and director Robert De Niro, and basketball star Michael Jordan. Even the Dixie Chicks have matching tattoos.

Although you must be at least eighteen years old to obtain a tattoo in most states, tattooing has become especially popular among young people. In the same 2003 Harrison poll, 13 percent of those tattooed were between the ages of eighteen and twenty-four years old.[2]

Choices that once made people appear to be courting the fringe of society are now commonplace. Today, it's not uncommon to see someone with multiple ear piercing or earlobes stretched to accommodate an eyelet. Tattoos appear on young and old alike across the entire United States, etched on arms, legs, backs, buttocks, hands, feet, necks, and faces. As these modifications have become increasingly sought after, it is now challenging to find a body modification that stands out from the crowd or expresses an avant-garde aesthetic. This search often moves people to seek more extreme forms of body modification. Some people attempt innovative designs or combinations of piercing and/or tattoos. Others opt for unusual, unconventional modifications such as cutting (scarification as adornment), branding (searing flesh with high heat in artistic patterns), or implantations (metal or plastic objects placed just under the skin to make visible impressions). Another recent trend is the popularity of mouth jewelry, or "grills," that are custom fitted to sit atop a person's teeth.

BE YOURSELF

No matter where your personal taste lies, many people who desire body modifications do so to emulate others. For teens, this often means mimicking their favorite celebrities. When you identify with the style of an artist's work or appreciate the fashion style of a pop icon, it's easy to fall into patterns of imitating his or her style. (The boom in belly button rings that followed Britney Spears's rise in popularity is just one example.)

In some cases, these choices act as a sort of shorthand when choosing friends and social groups. We've all experienced it: Someone passes us in the halls wearing a concert T-shirt or doodling the lyrics to a favorite song in class and we are instantly alerted to our shared interests. It's a natural way of developing a circle of friends.

It's comforting to meet like-minded people, especially in such an emotionally volatile time, but it's just as important to be true to yourself. Making a decision to permanently alter your body is a serious one. You should never get a tattoo or piercing as a way to fit in or try out a passing style or trend. Resist peer pressure if you can. Just because your favorite singer has a barbell through his or her nose and a brand on his or her arm, it doesn't mean it's the right choice for you. Even if you're the last member of your clique to get a tattoo, it's important to consider your individual values and personal goals beforehand. Take to heart the popular saying "your body is your temple" and keep in mind that you only get one body when navigating the decision about whether or not to permanently decorate it. The first step in making a wise decision about whether or not to get a modification is to be well informed about the benefits and risks associated with it.

WHAT IS BODY MODIFICATION?

Any change made to one's body for spiritual, fashion, social, or personal reasons may be referred to as body modification. This umbrella term includes piercing, tattooing, earlobe stretching, branding, and cutting, as well as more unusual choices such as dental, facial, or breast implants. Even dramatic and life-changing procedures such as gender-reassignment surgery fall into the body modification category.

People around the world have been adorning their bodies with a variety of body modifications since the earliest Egyptian dynasties. Although the style and frequency with which they're done so varies, there are commonalities shared by many cultures, some of which are still practiced today.

PIERCING

There is abundant evidence to suggest that body modification was a mode of self-expression and identification even in ancient times. Artifacts left by early peoples and found by archaeologists have led them to believe that this is the case. The University of Pennsylvania Museum of Archaeology and Anthropology showcased such evidence in a recent exhibit called "Bodies of Cultures: A World Tour of Body Modification." Museum curators made a special effort to explore the similarities between the body modifications of ancient peoples and those of today. The exhibit included a Mesopotamian carving of a man with multiple ear piercings dating back to 2900 BC. Other portions of the exhibit included Greek and Roman earrings from the fourth century AD, and earplugs and spools from Guatemala that date back to AD 900. These spools and plugs (used to stretch pierced earlobes) "have an amazing resemblance to those worn by the people of ancient Mexico,"[3] according to Elizabeth Straw, curator of the university's exhibit. Viewers hip to the body modifications of today will recognize them as similar to contemporary plugs and grommets.

Most of us can relate to ancient peoples who pierced the soft part of their earlobes. American women commonly had both of their ears pierced up until the 1920s, when they instead opted to keep their ears whole and wear clip-on earrings, which had become fashionable. It wasn't until the 1960s that single-ear piercing on each lobe enjoyed resurgence. In the 1970s, it became common for teenage girls to pierce both ears, a trend that continues. More than 85 percent of today's American women have singly pierced ears, as do many men. Many parents take young girls, and sometimes even infants, to have their ears pierced. What was once considered a racy body modification has now become part of mainstream culture.

Ear piercing remains a low-risk, inexpensive, and accessible body modification. The procedure, once only available in a doctor's office, is now performed at shopping malls, department stores, and salons in cities and towns across the country. It is now fairly common for people to opt for a second (or third or more) piercing, stacked on the outer lobe or pierced through the cartilage on the upper or inner parts of the ear. In fact, as early as 1999, *USA Today* cited the

Journal on Clinical Nursing Research, saying, "Fifteen to 25 percent of college-age students have some kind of body modification in the form of a tattoo or nontraditional piercing."[4]

According to Buzz McClain of the *Washington Post*, nontraditional piercing has enjoyed a long history. In a 2003 article, McClain briefly traced the history of body piercing back to the ancient Egyptians. He wrote, "Ancient Egyptian royalty pierced their navels, Roman centurions pierced their nipples, and American Indians used piercing in coming-of-age rituals."[5]

Nostril piecing is mentioned in the Bible's Old Testament, and it is still common in some Middle Eastern and South Asian cultures. In India, women typically have their left nostril pierced, a practice believed to ease the pain associated with childbirth. In the Americas, ancient Aztecs and Mayans, specifically shamans, sometimes had their tongues pierced because they believed that it would help them communicate with their gods. In these Mesoamerican cultures, people also pierced their lips, a practice called labret piercing, as a way to indicate social standing.

The contemporary trend of navel piercing in the West appears to have originated on the catwalk. In 1994, supermodel Christy Turlington arrived at a London fashion show sporting a navel ring. According to McClain in the *Washington Post*, "The next day, Naomi Campbell, apparently in a case of supermodel envy, made an appearance wearing a gold navel ring with a pearl fastener."[6] History was made. Assorted other celebrities and pop stars, like Madonna, Cher, and Janet Jackson, followed suit. Before long, plenty of women had also begun to indulge in the navel-piercing trend. Today, their numbers are countless. According to Bethra Szumski, president of the Association of Professional Piercers, determining an exact number would be "impossible," but she adds, business is "booming."[7]

THE RISE OF TATTOOING

Similarly, the current interest in tattooing as a cultural expression has ancient roots. Indigenous people the world over have included tattooing, piercing, stretching, scarring, and other forms of body modification in their coming-of-age rituals, to indicate their social standing, to identify themselves, and to express their religious or spiritual views.

Anthropologists have for many years correlated the ancient act of scarring and piercing with religion. "Whether it's a Buddhist lama drawing a blade across his tongue, a Lakota warrior hanging for hours by hooks puncturing his chest, or a sadhu [yogi] piercing his cheeks and tongue with small spears, nearly every culture has a sect that regards physical suffering, or an apparent indifference to it, as just another step in physical development,"[8] said Mark Hawthorne, in *Hinduism Today*.

Tattooing, believed to have started by cutting or puncturing the skin to achieve scarring, was a way in which participants could show their adoration to certain gods. In some cultures, anthropologists theorize, this voluntary endurance of pain was a way to express spiritual devotion. Egyptian artifacts believed to be funerary figures often have dot-and-dash tattoos like those found on female mummies of the same period.[9] Later Egyptian tattoos featured images of popular gods such as Bes, the Egyptian goddess of fertility.

Instruments likely used for tattooing date back to the Paleolithic era (38,000 BC to 10,000 BC) and were found on a variety of European archaeological digs. In 1991, archaeologists found the preserved frozen body of a man living more than 5,000 years ago on a mountain between Austria and Italy. Known as Ötzi the Iceman, he had more than fifty charcoal markings, some on the inside of his left knee, a series of straight lines above his kidneys, and another series of lines on his ankles. "Black lines on [his] back and ankles appear to be tattoos,"[10] wrote Bob Cullen in *Smithsonian Magazine*. Scientists are unsure if the tattoos were created for personal reasons, though some speculate that since the marks were placed on areas where X-rays revealed bone damage, they may have been applied to the skin to relieve pain.

Ancient Romans at first banned tattoos with the exception of branding criminals, but over time, their attitudes changed and soldiers in particular embraced tattoos as symbols of battles won or lost.

Katherine Dauge-Roth, an author and professor at Maine's Bowdoin College, discovered that Europeans practiced tattooing during the fifteenth century. In her research, she learned that England's religious pilgrims sometimes received tattoos of crosses on their skin to indicate they had made a journey to Bethlehem. According to Dauge-Roth, "The cross was not only a permanent souvenir of their voyage to Palestine and a way to show their religious zeal, but a sign that guaranteed their safe passage home. They write of experiences where, captured by bandits, they rolled up their sleeves, and, once recognized as [Christian] pilgrims, were set free, only having to pay a fee."[11] Similarly, medieval Christian crusaders had crosses tattooed on their bodies so if they died, they would be given a Christian burial. European sailors were also known to have crosses tattooed on their backs to prevent flogging. Religious and spiritual symbols have a long history of being tattooed on the skin, particularly in South Asia.

Tattoos were used as identifiers in other ways, too. While doing research at the archives of the Bibliothèque Nationale in Paris, France, Dauge-Roth located documents that suggested that tattooing was also used by the French government to condemn people for minor crimes. "In a time before fingerprinting," she says, "people condemned for crimes like minor theft, begging, counterfeiting, and smuggling were branded with letters specific to their crime: for instance, V for *voleur* (thief); M for *mendiant* (beggar)."[12]

POLYNESIAN CULTURES

The word "tattoo" is Polynesian in origin. It comes from the word *tatau* (meaning to mark or strike), which is used in Tahiti, Tonga, and Samoa.[13] In fact, the process of tattooing in Samoa has changed very little from that of 2,000 years ago, when young male Samoans were typically tattooed from their torso to their knees as a rite of passage into adulthood. The process of making the intricate traditional designs known as *pe'a* often took as long as three months, followed by several months of bathing in salt water and receiving massages to remove pathogens and promote healing.

In Hawaii, where there is a long history of imprinting the skin, the word *tatau* became *kakau*.[14] Hawaiians have tattooed their skin for centuries, often to commemorate major life events or to signify a spiritual connection to a god or a person, like to mark the death of a family member. For instance, in the 1820s, Hawaiian queen Ka'ahumanu, who bore tattoos on her legs and the palm of her left hand, had a tattoo engraved on her tongue as a mark of reverence for her deceased mother-in-law. When asked about the pain of the procedure, she replied, "*He eha nui no, he nui roa ra ku'u aroha*" ("Great pain indeed, [but] greater is my affection").[15] It's a Hawaiian custom to have three dots tattooed on the tongue as a symbol of mourning.

Nineteenth-century explorers to Hawaii also noted men tattooed on one side of their bodies, a solid black design called *pahupahu.*[16] Sometimes Hawaiian prisoners were even tattooed on the insides of their eyelids. In other cases, Hawaiians tattooed themselves for protection. For instance, a tattooed ring of dots around the ankle was believed to protect a person from a shark attack.[17]

THE MAORI

The act of tattooing came to New Zealand's Maori culture from Polynesia. According to Maori mythology, tattooing first appeared during a love affair between a young man by the name of Mataora (meaning "face of vitality") and a princess of the underworld named Niwareka, so it is no surprise that the Maori are best known for their full facial tattoos called *moko*.

Moko designs indicated a person's social class. In addition to the face, Maori women were commonly tattooed on the arms, legs, and sometimes groin. Like in all Polynesian cultures, these tattoos were applied by hand, with a chisel called an *uhi*, which punctured tiny holes in the skin. Blood was continually wiped away and replaced by pigment, which was rubbed into the skin to make the designs permanent. Today, the Maori still wear moko, the traditional designs that became popular again in the 1980s, though they now use modern techniques to apply them.

Not every culture has adopted modern methods. Some cultures still create tattoos by hand in a process similar to the one used by the Maori.

For instance, traditional Japanese tattoos called *irezumi* are hand-poked with sharpened bamboo or steel needles. Once the ancient distinction of criminals, Japanese tattooing became a part of the wider culture around 1700. The tiny holes are then filled with ink or ashes to outline the designs, which are often full-body images. Interestingly, however, these full-body designs are now considered dangerous. People who have a large percentage of their skin covered by tattoos are known to have shorter life spans.[18]

"[Full-body tattooing] is a form of self-destruction; fully tattooed people live shorter lives because their skin can't breathe properly and some of the inks are poisonous," said Diane Ackerman in *A Natural History of the Senses*.[19]

TATTOOING INFLUENCES EUROPEANS

News of tattooing made its way west during the European age of exploration. In 1691, English explorer William Dampier brought a tattooed man back from the South Pacific to England. The tattooed man, Jeoly, became known as the Painted Prince and was placed on exhibit, fascinating anyone who took notice.[20]

Nearly a century later, in 1769, English explorer Captain James Cook, during one of several voyages to the Polynesian Islands, "discovered" tattooing in Tahiti and cleverly documented it for Europeans. Cook's expedition artist Sydney Parkinson did a variety of detailed drawings of tattoos on the islanders, finally introducing Europeans to the word "tattoo" as it is used today.[21]

Nicholas Thomas, professor of anthropology at Goldsmiths College, University of London, and consultant for a 2002 exhibit about the history of tattooing at London's Maritime Museum, noted the impact of the Polynesian cultures on European society. He said in *Time* magazine, "Tattooing is an example of how a small, remote society had a tremendously significant impact on European culture. [The introduction of tattooing] changed the bodies of Europeans in a radical way."[22] According to Thomas, European sailors were immediately taken with the practice. A sailor's tattoos acted as a sort of visual résumé detailing his accomplishments. For example, a bird on a sailor's chest meant he had crossed the ocean. Two birds meant a sailor had sailed across the ocean and back. A turtle meant he had crossed the equator. Many sailors kept a running list of ports where they had worked by tattooing their names on their lower legs or upper arms. Penalties for falsifying one's reputation by adding tattoos that hadn't been earned were severe.

Native Americans were also tattooed. Seventeenth-century English writer William Strachey described the men and women of the Powhatan tribes he encountered in the coastal region that is now Virginia:

> [They] have their armes, breasts, thighes, shoulders, and faces, cuningly

> ymbrodered with divers workes, for pouncing or searing their skyns with a kind of instument heated in the fier. They figure therin flowers and fruits of sondry lively kinds, as also snakes, serpents . . . this they doe by dropping uppon the seared flesh sondry coulers, which, rub'ed into the stampe, will never be taken awaye agayne, because yt will not only be dryed into the flesh, but grow therein.[23]

The first written records of tattooing in America are found in logs kept by ship captains. In America's early days, tattoos were the territory of sailors and travelers almost exclusively, though tattooing soon became highly popular among U.S. Navy sailors and Civil War soldiers. "Thousands of men were tattooed on the battlefields. Martin Hildebrandt, one of the first American tattooers of record, was a migrant battlefield tattooer. Being indifferent to politics, he ran back and forth from the Confederate and Union sides, setting up shop wherever the trade was best,"[24] said writer Mike McCabe. During the nineteenth century, tattoo culture grew throughout U.S. port districts and continued spreading into America's cities.

THE MACHINE AGE

Before the invention of electricity, getting a tattoo was a slow, painful process. Before the 1890s, tattoos were applied by hand with a single needle and generally one color of ink. The process was excruciating. There were only a handful of tattoo artists in the country, and each of them were highly sought after.

In 1876, Thomas Edison patented an engraving device he called the autographic printer, an unsuccessful invention that was converted into the first tattoo machine, the "electric engraving pen,"[25] by New York tattoo artist Samuel O'Reilly in 1891. The new machine, which O'Reilly used in his downtown New York tattoo shop located among the dime museums and beer halls in Chatham Square, could inject ink into tiny punctures it made on the skin's surface. Twenty days after O'Reilly filed his patent, an Englishman named Thomas Riley filed a patent for a variation of the machine, making the process of applying a tattoo much faster and less painful. Still a far cry from the efficient machines of today, they made the process tolerable enough that some of the more adventurous socialites of the day got tattoos.

Early tattoo aficionados who were not as wealthy took jobs in traveling circuses and sideshows as "painted men" or "tattooed ladies" to support their interest. The most elaborately decorated men and women were often the most sought after. Many were paid high salaries, some as much as $200 per week [or about $3,000 today],[26] as they were constantly in demand by rival circuses, many of which also hired tattoo artists to travel along with the show.

Word of tattooing spread and a small number of people pioneered what is today's body modification culture. In addition to sailors and circus performers, some daring socialites indulged in body modification, including Lady Randolph Churchill, mother of Prime Minister Winston Churchill, who had a snake tattooed around her left wrist as a "bracelet."[27]

Very slowly, the numbers of people with tattoos increased. Until the 1940s, tattoos primarily remained among the interests of military men and people on the fringe of society. During World War II, however, it became more common for American soldiers to get tattoos to commemorate their wartime experiences. The sight of returning veterans with colorful tattoos of exotic places helped make tattooing more acceptable.

During the early days, most people considered tattooing as a way of marking the body with visual clues that told a story, much like a scrapbook. "[T]attooing, from the end of World War I through the late 1960s or early 1970s, was chiefly souvenir shopping; one marked the body the way people used to put travel stickers on their suitcases. Ports of call, hearts (broken and otherwise), sailing ships, girls in grass skirts, mermaids, sea monsters, [or] pirates. And there were always religious tattoos—twenty percent of all tattoos are religious," said author John Irving.[28]

TATTOO CULTURE

Although the 1950s ushered in a new appreciation for the bohemian lifestyle with the rise of beat poets like Jack Kerouac and Allen Ginsberg, tattooing remained limited in its exposure. It was during the 1960s and 1970s that tattooing really took its place in mainstream society. Lyle Tuttle was right in the middle of this movement and he has since become its icon. In an interview in *Prick* magazine, Tuttle described getting his first tattoo in San Francisco in 1946:

> I was able to take a Greyhound bus down to the big city [where] I ran across an old tattoo shop. I'd seen servicemen with tattoos and to me it was symbolic of an adventure and that's what I was on. It meant you'd been over the horizon . . . I stumbled and mumbled and looked around and saw a heart on the wall with the word mother on it. It was $3.50. I pointed and said, "That one." Man, he had that thing on me so quick . . . I just couldn't believe it.[29]

In 1960, Tuttle opened a small studio in San Francisco called Lyle Tuttle Tattoo, above a Greyhound bus station. He said it was the spirit of the times that made society ripe for a tattoo revolution:

> Women's liberation put tattooing back on the map. With women getting a newfound freedom, they could get tattooed if they so desired. It increased and opened the market by 50 percent of the population . . . For three years, I tattooed almost nothing but women [who] made tattooing a softer and kinder art form.[30]

Tuttle was in the right place at the right time. San Francisco in the 1960s was a hotbed for progressive thinking and revolutionary counterculture. One way the youth of the time expressed themselves about the war in Vietnam, the civil rights movement, and the sexual revolution was to get tattooed. Throughout the decade, tattoos appeared on hippies and revolutionaries, many of whom later helped usher body art into mainstream society. Today, a Tuttle tattoo is quite sought after and highly admired, since he is considered the father of modern tattooing.

Meanwhile, in New York City, health officials blamed an outbreak of hepatitis B on tattoo artists in 1961 and the practice of tattooing was outlawed there for thirty-five years. (When the ban was finally lifted in 1997, more than 200 tattoo artists applied for licensing in New York during the first twelve months.) The 1961 ruling led to a ban on tattooing in many other cities across America, even though there was no distinct proof that the outbreak was linked to New York's tattoo parlors.

In the late 1970s and early 1980s, the punk movement embraced body modification in an effort to mock bourgeois society, popularizing multiple ear piercing and visible tattoos, especially among youths in England and the United States. Earrings became more common on men. Multiple piercing was no longer shocking. It was not uncommon to see people of either gender with a row of earrings all along the outer line of their ear. Even the innocuous safety pin took on new meaning. According to authors Patricia Anne Cunningham and Susan Voso Lab in their book *Dress and Popular Culture*, "The punk's safety pin through the cheek shocks the typical observer because the symbolic use and meaning of a safety pin has nothing to do with self-mutilation. Indeed, it is meant to protect the body, and is often associated with harmless babies."[31] Like symbolic tribal associations made through the identification of certain marks on the body, punks identified each other by certain tattoos and piercings. But it was during the 1990s that body modification moved away from the fringe and into the mainstream.

In the 1990s, piercings and tattoos showed up on pop stars, professional athletes, and almost everyone in between. On young women, pierced tongues and belly buttons became popular. Pierced ears, noses, and eyebrows appeared on young men. Even Rachel and Phoebe on the television hit *Friends* made a trip to a tattoo parlor. The craze was on. In 2006, the *San Diego Union-Tribune* cited a 2004 Harris poll claiming that "thirty-four percent of Americans thought tattoos made them appear sexy and 29 percent thought they made them more attractive."[32]

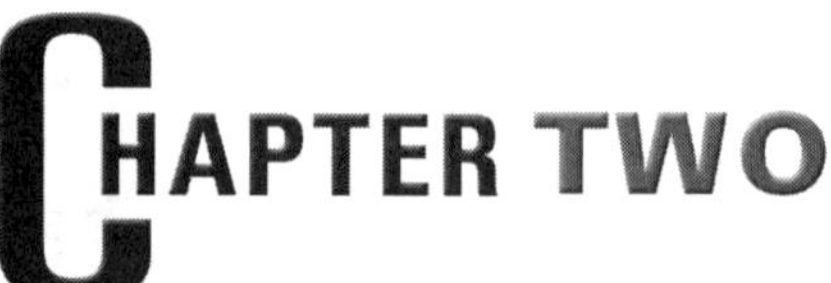

Chapter Two

What Are the Health Risks?

Because applying a tattoo breaks the skin, there are a variety of risks associated with the process, including contracting blood-borne diseases, skin infections or disorders, and allergic reactions.

If you're thinking you'd like to join the growing number of Americans whose bodies have been inked and/or pierced, there is a great deal to learn about the health risks associated with your options.

All body modification involves some damage to and healing of the body to complete the process. When considering your options, it's important to learn as much as possible about the modification itself, how it heals, and how you should care for it. Gathering reliable information from reputable sources is a crucial part of making a responsible decision to obtain body art.

TATTOOS

A tattoo is a permanent marking created by making a series of small puncture wounds, about one-eighth of an inch into the skin, with a needle or group of needles.

Tattoo artists should be willing to discuss this process with you and answer any questions that you may have before you decide to go ahead with the procedure. You should seek tattoos only from fully trained and licensed tattoo artists. Also, anyone seeking a tattoo should first obtain a hepatitis B vaccination to safeguard against the spread of one form of this dangerous virus.

At the beginning of your session, you will be asked to show a photo identification to prove you are at least eighteen years of age and sign consent forms saying that you are healthy and not under the influence of drugs or alcohol. If you are underage, most tattoo artists will not work on you. Others may if you have a parent or guardian with you or a parent or guardian gives you written permission.

You and your artist will discuss your tattoo, the process, and your design. Because laws governing licensed tattoo artists vary by state, these rules may be different depending on where you live. You may want to look at flash (tattoo designs) in the studio or you may have your own original idea for a tattoo.

Once everything is agreed upon, the tattoo artist will generally transfer the outline of the design onto your skin. Some artists suggest living with this drawn-on design for a few days as a test run for the permanent marking.

Any tattoo session begins with the artist washing his or her hands before cleaning the area of skin that will be tattooed. Wearing surgical gloves and occasionally covering his or her mouth and nose with a surgical mask, the artist then opens a sterile, single-use needle, which is inserted into the tattoo machine. (If the artist does not open the needle in front of you, then it may not be sterile. If this is the case, you should leave the shop immediately.)

All equipment used for the tattooing procedure should be sterilized in an autoclave—a machine specifically designed to sterilize medical tools and instruments. Using the tattoo machine, the artist begins to etch the outline of the tattoo into your skin. As the outline is completed, it is washed with soap and water. Any blood on the surface of the skin will be cleaned with a disposable towel.

Having completed the outline, the artist will open another set of sterile, single-use needles for filling out the design with colors. Smaller tattoos can sometimes be completed in only one forty-five-minute session, but larger, more complicated tattoos may have to be completed in a series of sessions, each scheduled approximately four weeks apart. When the session is completed, the artist will wipe any blood away with a disposable towel and bandage the skin.

HEALTH RISKS OF TATTOOING

Because applying a tattoo breaks the skin, there are a variety of risks associated with the process, including contracting blood-borne diseases, skin infections or disorders, and allergic reactions.

Blood-borne diseases such as HIV (the virus that causes AIDS), hepatitis C, hepatitis B, tuberculosis, and tetanus can all be transmitted by coming into contact with the blood of an infected person. Licensed tattoo artists are required by law to use only single-use needles to guard against the transmission of these diseases, but there is still some risk associated with coming into contact with equipment that is used to tattoo hundreds, if not thousands, of people.

In fact, a 2001 study by the University of Texas Southwestern Medical Center suggested that there might be a correlation in the United States between the rise of popularity in tattoos and the increase in hepatitis C infections. Out of 600 patients surveyed, 22 percent who had tattoos were infected with hepatitis versus a 3.5 percent infection rate of those without tattoos.[1] The study further urges physicians to screen their tattooed patients for hepatitis C. According to Robert Haley, MD, and coauthor of the study, "As far as I know, Texas is the only state that inspects tattoo parlors, even though hepatitis C can give you a fatal disease that can cut your life short by 20 or 30 years."[2]

It is now widely believed that people with tattoos are nine times more likely to be infected with hepatitis C than non-tattooed individuals.

Getting a tattoo can in some cases lead to a variety of bacterial infections, some of which can be life-threatening. According to the Centers for Disease Control and Prevention (CDC), some of the more serious skin infections associated with tattooing are on the rise. Health writers for Reuters reported in June 2006 that six recent outbreaks of the "superbug" methicillin-resistant *Staphylococcus aureus* (MRSA) had been traced to unlicensed tattoo artists in Kentucky, Ohio, and Vermont.[3] According to Reuters, "MRSA infection typically manifests in abscesses or areas of inflammation on the skin, though it can also lead to more serious problems such as pneumonia, blood infections, or in some cases, necrotizing fasciitis, also referred to as the 'flesh-eating disease.'"[4] The outbreaks affected more than forty people, thirty-four of whom had gotten a tattoo from an unlicensed artist, possibly due to equipment that had not been properly disinfected. Signs of skin infection may include redness, irritation, warmth, swelling, and a pus-like discharge. If you see any of these signs on or around your new tattoo, you should seek immediate help from a medical professional.

Other risks of getting tattooed include skin disorders such as tiny bumps forming around the design called granulomas, especially if your tattoo includes red ink. Raised scar tissue can also form from tattooing the skin. Red ink is also the cause of many allergic reactions. In a 2005 issue of *Dermatology Times*, Dr. Anne E. Lanmann, MD, stated that 13 percent of recently tattooed youth had experienced healing problems associated with tattoos done outside a professional salon and those that included red ink.[5]

You should never get tattooed with india ink because it contains poison that can make you ill. The poison from india ink can also remain in your body and, in females, possibly contribute to birth defects in children born years later.

Finally, the iron in some tattoo inks can be pulled out of the skin during an MRI (magnetic resonance imaging, a medical procedure that scans the body to examine internal organs). The ink can also obscure the image produced by an MRI and therefore hinder medical management.

TATTOO AFTERCARE

In order to fight infection or further injury to the area, the bandage must stay on a fresh tattoo for at least twenty-four hours. During that time, it is important not to scratch the skin, or pick at any scabs that might form. While scabs may look like an obstruction of the tattoo, they are only temporary and are an important part of the healing process. Picking at the scab can cause infection and scarring that may alter the design of the tattoo.

Any redness or swelling of the newly tattooed area might be soothed with the application of an ice pack. Other care will include washing the area with antibacterial soap and applying antibacterial ointments. Use soaps and ointments recommended and/or provided by your tattoo artist. Chemicals such as hydrogen peroxide and rubbing alcohol are not recommended for soothing or cleaning tattooed skin.

For a period of two weeks, your new tattoo might look glossy; this is a sign that the skin has not completely healed. In tattoo culture, this is called "fresh ink." Until that glossy look fades and the tone of the tattooed area begins to match the rest of your skin, it will require special care. Never get another tattoo before this condition fades.

Personal or aesthetic risks involved with tattooing are that the design may change over time. Additionally, not all inks are visible with all skin tones. For instance, people with darker skin might be disappointed in the effects of colored inks. Changes in the skin over time from aging or stretching during pregnancy or from weight gain or loss will also change your tattoo. Discuss inks and design durability with a tattoo artist before making a final decision on where you have decided to place your tattoo.

It's possible that your feelings about your tattoo will change over time as your tastes mature. For example, you may not want a girlfriend's or a boyfriend's name tattooed on your body after you part ways. Or, as you enter college, you may wish you hadn't had your high school mascot tattooed on your arm. If ever you want to get a corporate job or join the military, you may wish you hadn't gotten a gang tattoo.

TATTOO REMOVAL

Never make a hasty decision to get a tattoo because you think that you can have it removed. While it is true that tattoos can be removed, it is important to remember that the process is very expensive, quite painful, and does not leave the skin with a flawless appearance. In addition, some tattoo inks are more difficult to remove than others.

Tattoos are most often removed by laser surgery, a procedure performed by a dermatologic surgeon on an outpatient basis with local anesthesia. This means that you won't need to stay overnight for the procedure and that the anesthesia will numb only the area where the tattoo is located. However, the surgery can be painful depending on the extent of the tattoo removal and the color of inks that were used to create it. Laser surgery is costly. A small tattoo that cost less than $100 to obtain might cost between $1,500 and $2,000 to remove, depending on the number of laser treatments needed.

Dermabrasion is another treatment to remove tattoos. In this procedure, a surgeon "sands" the skin so that its surface and middle layers are removed. He or she then uses a combination of surgical and dressing techniques to help raise and absorb the ink in the skin.

Surgical excision is the third option in which a surgeon literally removes the tattoo with a scalpel and closes the wound with stitches. This method allows complete removal and always leaves a scar.

An alternative to tattoo removal is "inking over" an unwanted tattoo with a darker tattoo, leaving a denser, more intense-looking design.

HEALTH RISKS OF PIERCING

Any time the skin is broken, a person risks infection. The same risk holds true when you choose to get your body pierced. A piercing is simply a hole poked through soft body tissue with a needle and then fitted with appropriate jewelry. Although you might know of friends who have done their piercing themselves or had a piercing done by a friend, these practices are not safe. The use of piercing kits is considered extremely risky. In a 2005 study by the American Association of Piercers, the use of piercing kits has been linked to an increased risk of infection and disease transmission.[6] Anyone who wants to obtain a piercing should do so only from a licensed professional. According to the Association of Professional Piercers, only forty-three states currently have legislation "regarding personal criteria for the piercer, requirements for the piercing establishment, and highly specific laws necessitating parental consent for the piercing of minors."[7]

Before deciding to get a piercing, you'll need to choose your body jewelry. While trendy and inexpensive body jewelry is available at shopping malls and fashion jewelry counters, it's best to buy your jewelry from your piercer. They can help you decide which styles and gauges (width of wires) are appropriate for the placement and size of your piercing. They will also be more likely to carry quality metals that won't cause an allergic reaction as your piercing heals. Suggested metals include surgical steel, solid 14-karat or 18-karat gold, niobium, titanium, or platinum.

Just like the forms you sign when you request a tattoo, you will have to sign paperwork stating that you are of age to be pierced and that you consent to the procedure. You will be asked to show identification with your photo, and if you are under eighteen years old, your parent or guardian will need to be present or provide permission in writing.

A small mark will be drawn on your skin where the piercing will be placed. The person doing the piercing will then wash his or her hands and the area of your body to be pierced before opening a small, sterile packet containing a single-use, stainless-steel needle. Some needles are used by hand and others are inserted into a piercing gun; the method depends on the placement of the piercing. All equipment should be sterilized in an autoclave. The person doing the piercing then makes the puncture wound and immediately slips the jewelry through the hole before washing away any blood. Depending on the location of the wound, the process is relatively painless, though certain spots are more sensitive than others. Some areas also take much longer to heal, like naval and nipple areas.

"Doctors say that tongue and genital piercings can also provide channels for bacteria and viruses to enter the bloodstream after the piercing procedure,"[8] according to a 2005 article in the *New York Times*. Given this information, people who are pierced are constantly exposed to the risks of infection. In addition, genital piercing can increase the risks of sexually transmitted diseases such as HPV (human papillomavirus) and HIV, since they are prone to break condoms and tear flesh, further exposing a person to infection and potentially infectious body fluids.[9]

Piercing through the tongue makes people especially vulnerable to infection spreading from the mouth through the bloodstream or the tissues of the neck. Experts have traced deadly infections of the vital organs back to tongue piercings. This is why doctors advise people, especially those with existing heart problems, to take antibiotics prior to and immediately after undergoing some piercing procedures. Most people, however, don't consult their doctors as part of their decision-making process.

MYTHS AND FACTS ABOUT PIERCING AND TATTOOING

Myth: You can pierce your own body with an ice cube, a safety pin, and a potato.

Fact: Home piercing is unsafe and not recommended. Even the use of piercing kits carries a greater risk of infection and tearing than having your piercing done by a professional. Also, avoid having anything pierced (or tattooed) at potentially unlicensed establishments such as those featured at flea markets, carnivals, boardwalk venders, fairs, and similar facilities.

Myth: Gold is one of the safest metals for body jewelry.

Fact: Pure surgical metals, like steel and titanium, are much less likely to spark allergic reactions than gold. Nickel, which is an ingredient in some alloys used to make body jewelry, seems to cause allergic reactions more than other metals do.

Myth: Once you take your jewelry out, your piercing will heal over and disappear.

Fact: It is possible that your piercing will develop a keloid (a thick, raised scar) as it heals. If you stretch your piercing, you should remember that stretching may be permanent. Some people notice that their piercing closes up slightly, or entirely, when jewelry is removed, but this does not happen to all people.

Myth: A tattoo artist will tattoo any area of the body that you desire.

Fact: Many tattoo artists won't tattoo certain areas of the body, like the palms of the hands, the fingers, and the bottoms of the feet. Others have even more stringent restrictions, and some states have laws forbidding tattooing on certain parts of the body such as the face, near the eyes, or the fingertips. Check with your area artists for specific information.

Myth: Even though I just got a tattoo a few months ago, I can still donate blood during the annual blood drive at my school.

Fact: According to the American Red Cross, blood donors must wait at least twelve months after getting a tattoo before donating blood.

PIERCING AFTERCARE

The person who provided your piercing will likely discuss with you how to care for it and give you a sheet of paper with aftercare instructions. These generally include washing the area with antibacterial soap twice a day and possibly rinsing the area with salt water. Listen carefully: Getting a piercing can be overwhelming, and you may not fully remember all of the aftercare instructions when you get home. Just like when you get a tattoo, you should watch for signs of infection at the piercing site, like redness, irritation, swelling, warmth, or a puslike discharge. If you see any one of these signs, you should immediately consult a medical professional, since infections can travel through the bloodstream and become even more health-threatening. Depending on the location, a piercing can take several months to a year to heal. If you are concerned about a long healing time, discuss various piercing locations and expected healing rates with a professional.

The *Journal of the American Medical Association* (JAMA) warns that improperly cleaned piercing equipment or jewelry can carry contaminations and lead to serious infections such as hepatitis.[10] It recommends seeking fully trained piercers who use sterile, single-use equipment and have stringent cleaning policies. It also suggests that piercing guns are riskier than other means of piercing.

According to a 2005 article in the *New York Times*,

> New laws regulating piercing [in Oregon] were drafted in response to an outbreak of an antibiotic-resistant strain of the bacterium *Pseudomonas aeruginosa* in ear cartilage. Health officials traced [the outbreak] to a piercing gun at a jewelry kiosk. Four people were hospitalized; permanent ear deformities, including the removal of ear cartilage, resulted.[11]

The risk isn't over once the piercing session is finished. A medical study published in *Dermatology Times* states that of seventy-one participants in a study measuring complications of body modifications, specifically piercing, 18 percent of them had complications lasting two or more weeks. Twenty-three percent of people with a mouth piercing had chipped or broken teeth as a result of living with their body jewelry in place.[12] It is also possible that heavy-gauge body jewelry will tear the skin, ruining your piercing, and giving your previously pierced skin a torn or forked look.

According to Dr. Scott Hammer, professor of medicine at Columbia College of Physicians and Surgeons, "One piercing in ten becomes infected. *Staphylococcus* bacteria, which can live on the skin and in the nose, is a frequent cause."[13]

A piercing may close once the jewelry is removed, but this relies largely on the placement of the piercing, the gauge of the jewelry, the age of the piercing, and the body chemistry of the person being pierced. Many people develop a keloid, or raised and thickened scar tissue, over a piercing after removing jewelry. This is a natural part of the healing process, but some people find it unattractive.

TEN GREAT QUESTIONS TO ASK A BODY ART ARTIST

When deciding on an artist to help you achieve your body modification, you should always ask questions beforehand. While making up your mind, consider asking the tattoo artist or skilled piercer the following questions:

1. What type of training do you have?
2. Are you licensed by the state?
3. How often are your tools and instruments cleaned and sterilized?
4. Do you use single-use needles?
5. What type of inks do you use?
6. How are problems at this institution traced?
7. Whom do I contact if I have problems with my tattoo and/or piercing?
8. How should I care for my tattoo and/or piercing?
9. What type of metal will be used for my piercing?
10. How long will it take my tattoo and/or piercing to heal?

STRETCHING

Stretching is a prolonged and stylized method of piercing that results in the enlargement of a piercing or body part, usually the earlobes but occasionally the lips or other areas, for aesthetic, social, and/or spiritual reasons. (In some places, stretching is called "gauging," a reference to the increasing widths of metals placed in the ear to stretch it.) A stretched piercing is often maintained with grommetlike jewelry, tapers, weights, and/or plugs.

Of the body modification methods discussed in this chapter, stretching is the most time-consuming. It often requires months, sometimes years, of careful attention to develop into the desired shape.

For stretching, the piercing process is followed by months or maybe years of encouraging the hole and the surrounding area to increase in size. This is accomplished by inserting larger gauge jewelry into the piercing site, incrementally and over time. It is generally recommended that stretchers not increase the piercing site faster than one size per month.

Working with regulated jewelry is the best way to measure your stretching and monitor your process. Avoid using found objects to stretch your piercing because they can increase your chances of developing an infection. To ease the stretching process, use a water-based lubricant, or stretch after the heat from a shower or a hot compress has made your skin more pliable.

Other objects for stretching include tapers—horn-shaped objects made of metal, wood, glass, bone, or other safe materials that begin at a comfortable gauge and gradually increase in diameter. Some professionals use tapers as a tool for inserting larger jewelry into a piercing, but you might prefer to wear them as jewelry. Weights can also be used for stretching. Tiny metal weights are attached to the ear via a plug, or the piercing alone, so that they stretch the piercing.

Another way to achieve a stretched earlobe is by scalpelling, a process by which a professional cuts the lobe with a scalpel and then inserts a plug with a taper. No flesh is removed in this procedure. A dermal punch, a surgical instrument similar to a common paper hole punch, can also be used to remove some flesh of the soft earlobe to accommodate plugs. (A paper hole punch cannot achieve this look safely or effectively.)

Stretching too quickly can result in tearing and scarring, which will be painful, is likely to become infected, and may hinder your ability to achieve your desired modification. Quick stretching may also result in a "piercing blowout." A piercing blowout is when the skin of the ear grows over the jewelry. In this case, an unusual ridge of flesh, looking something like a lip, forms over the edge of the jewelry.

CHAPTER THREE

Different Modifications for Different People

THOSE WITH MULTIPLE PIERCINGS WERE MUCH MORE LIKELY TO HAVE EXPERIENCED STRESSFUL LIFE EVENTS SUCH AS A SEVERE INJURY OR ILL-NESS [OR] ABUSE OR DEATH OF A LOVED ONE.

Tattooing and body piercing involve a certain amount of pain, risk, expense, and social stigma. Having examined these processes in more detail, you may be thinking, "Right on, I can handle it; I'm on my way to the nearest salon," or "EEK! I feel faint; I don't think I could ever endure a body modification."

Some people think about getting a tattoo for years before actually doing so, while others might decide quickly.

It's also okay to think a tattoo or piercing is cool or interesting on other people but maybe not something you would do to your own body. People have chosen to be tattooed or pierced for any number of reasons. Some of those reasons may be yours; others might sound odd or irrational to you. Either way, getting a tattoo or body piercing is a personal choice and not one that should be taken lightly.

Recently, journalists, medical professionals, psychologists, and sociologists have conducted research aimed at discovering why body art has become so popular. They do this because they are interested in learning about changing attitudes in society.

Lynne Carroll and Roxanne Anderson conducted a study like this in 2002 and published their findings in the journal *Adolescence*. Searching for answers about why girls sought body modifications, the researchers interviewed seventy-nine girls between the ages of fifteen and seventeen and asked them questions about their body art.

Thirty-four girls in the study had nontraditional piercings, twenty-nine had their ears pierced, and sixteen had tattoos. According to the report, "Nine [girls] had pierced their tongues, nine had their navels pierced, six pierced their noses, three pierced above their eyebrows, and two indicated that their piercings were on another part of the body. Tattoo locations included legs (5), stomach (4), arms (3), breasts (2), shoulder (1), and hand (1)."[1] When asked about the reasons behind their body modifications, the researchers received simple answers. According to their results, "Thirteen [of the girls] stated they 'wanted it,' six stated it was 'in style,' four stated 'it was cute' . . . and one said 'it was fun.'"[2] When pressed for more specific reasons, most girls either directly indicated or indirectly implied that their choices were made as an assertion of their independence.

Other people may have more personal reasons for taking the plunge, but for many, the choice to get body art has more to do with specific experiences. For instance, in a 2004 study based on about 280 University of Florida graduates, researchers found that "those with multiple piercing were much more likely to have experienced stressful life events such as a severe injury or illness [or] abuse or death of a loved one."[3]

SELF-EXPRESSION

For the large number of those interested in expressing themselves by getting tattooed and/or pierced, there is now an active, engaging, and interesting community that has developed around people who respect and admire body modification. These people can be found on the Internet, in print publications, in businesses, in competitions, and at elaborate conventions. Interested people of all ages and walks of life meet and share ideas, stories, and experiences about their tattoos and piercings.

We all have a need to belong. Some of us satisfy that need in less conventional ways than others. For some people, getting a tattoo is a very personal, private decision, and for others, it's a rite of passage into adulthood. Still more people consider body modification an art form. In the following examples, more specific reasons for getting body art are discussed.

War Tattoos

Amy Krakow, author of *The Total Tattoo Book*, says the reasons for getting a tattoo "have always been threefold—love, loyalty, and bravado."[4] Perhaps this is the reason that during almost every American war, a large number of soldiers obtain tattoos as personal memorials to their experiences in conflict. This is a practice that has been ongoing since the Revolutionary War. Some people felt the calling after 9/11, while others got tattoos to remind them of troops we lost. Still more might get a tattoo to symbolize a loved one while he or she is away. One wartime favorite is a simple peace sign. Others get portraits, flags, and other patriotic designs.

In 1996, Cpl. Joseph Giardino, a twenty-three-year-old veteran of the Persian Gulf War, explained to *Wall Street Journal* reporter Michael M. Phillips that he had "Some Gave All" tattooed across his back in blue as a way of remembering his friends and fellow soldiers who died in the war. That same reporter quotes Lance Cpl. Kelly Miller who tattooed "Remember the Fallen" on his upper arm in honor of his squad leader who saved his life in battle. Phillips wrote, "Somehow, the needle's prick relieved the sorrow of loss and the guilt of survival."[5] He believes that the permanence of the memorial and the pain of getting the tattoo may have helped soldiers psychologically; others might say the pain of enduring a tattoo helps survivors deal with the guilt felt by losing friends and loved ones. Other soldiers agree. Phillips continues by quoting Sgt. Jason Liemeux: "When I was feeling the pain of the tattoo, it was actually making it OK that those guys got killed and I didn't."[6]

Gang Tattoos

Just like people in the military mark their bodies in symbolic tattoos, so do many gang members. Sometimes they get "official" tattoos to represent their membership in the gang, often a specific emblem or symbol. These highly visible markings are also a way of permanently separating gang members from mainstream society, since the tattoos often appear on the hands and face. In many cases, gang members themselves will tattoo other gang members, often in less than sanitary conditions. All members of a certain gang normally have the same, or very similar, markings, like a cross or three dots in a pyramid shape, often applied on the hand between the thumb and index finger. Other common markings are more fatalistic such as tombstones (sometimes used to denote years lost due to time spent in prison), "R.I.P." (Rest in Peace), symbolic numbers (sometimes a homage to deceased gang members), or phrases in a member's native language such as "my crazy life" or "I care for nothing."

Having similar tattoos is a way to identify with other gang members, but having visible gang tattoos can cause many problems. Just as the tattoo shows your membership in a particular gang, it will also mark you as an enemy of rival gang members. Plus, having a permanent mark linking you to a specific gang makes it difficult to leave that gang.

In 2005, the *Washington Post* reported on social service programs in the Washington, D.C., and Virginia areas that offer free tattoo removal for young people.[7] Programs like these often have age restrictions and require some community service in exchange for removal services, but for young people who regret their earlier affiliations with gangs, getting a tattoo removed is often a way to make a fresh start. Getting a gang tattoo removed also helps people get hired by employers who would think twice before considering someone who was affiliated with a gang.

According to *Washington Post* reporter David Cho, one man in the tattoo removal program was a nineteen-year-old from Richmond, Virginia, who had been a gang member for five years. After spending some time in prison after robbing a store while he was in the Bloods, he wanted to start over and join the armed services. The problem was that he couldn't join the Army with his gang markings, the words "THUG LIFE" tattooed just below his knuckles. According to the article, "He realized the shallowness of the group while in prison"[8] and wanted to avoid association with and retribution from other gang members. The tattoo removal program allowed him to start over.

People who have gang tattoos should be aware that several states, including California and Florida, now maintain active databases filled with photographs of tattoos featured on the bodies of people who have been arrested. They use this information to aid them in identifying gang affiliations and their associated markings.

Family Tattoos

Former President Theodore Roosevelt had a tattoo of the Roosevelt family crest, and his daughter, Alice, was tattooed as well. Another popular choice for tattoos is the name of a parent, spouse, or child, made as marks of love and devotion.

"I'd rather do my children's names than, say, a girlfriend's,"[9] remarked one pierced and tattooed man. "My girlfriend may leave me, and then I wouldn't want the tattoo anymore, but my children will always be my children. Nothing will change that. I could tattoo their names on my arm and feel good about it."

People occasionally tattoo the name of a deceased relative on their bodies as a memorial. A permanent tattoo seems to offer people a way to feel OK about living even after their loved one is gone, and it is a way to have their loved one with them permanently. When they're missing that person, they can be reminded of their deep connection by looking at their tattoo.

Survival Tattoos

Tattooing is becoming a popular way for cancer survivors to memorialize their struggle with the disease. An example of this would be the women who, after having a breast removed in a mastectomy, tattoo beautiful images over the scars from their surgery. It is a way of making themselves beautiful, celebrating their bravery, and of showing solidarity with other women who've had similar experiences. When they look at their chests after the surgery and the tattoo, they see more than a body that was modified beyond their control, but one modified by choice. Getting a tattoo after a mastectomy can be a healthy way to reclaim and reconnect with one's body.

In 2006, the *Seattle Times* ran a story about a woman named Jackie Floyd who had her chest tattooed after a radical mastectomy. Describing her reasons for having butterflies and flowers tattooed over her surgical scars, Floyd told the reporter, "The loss and the renewal needed to be in the same space. I wanted an image of what I was going to do."[10] Floyd regained control of her body by having her scars made beautiful through the act of tattooing.

Religious Tattoos

Many people obtain tattoos for religious or cultural reasons. In some native cultures and religions, rituals are associated with tattooing, piercing, and even scarification. In some cases, getting a tattoo may signify the beginning of adulthood. Piercing might be part of a vision quest. There are as many variants on religious themes as there are cultures and traditions in the world.

In contemporary American culture, people may wear a tattoo of a spiritual symbol such as a cross or a quote from scripture as a way to show commitment to their religious choices or to identify with other members of the same religion. Christians might have crucifixes or saints tattooed on their arms. Similarly, people who practice Eastern religions might have yin/yang symbols or other meaningful designs. People interested in Wicca might have pentagrams, fairies, or other symbols of nature tattooed on them. These tattoos have great significance for the tattooed, but clergy and other religious leaders are divided when asked about body modifications.

Some orthodox or conservative religious groups frown upon body modification. They believe that people were created in the image of God and shouldn't change their appearance in a way that is permanent. This is especially true for those who practice Judaism, for the Torah reads, "Ye shall not make any cuttings in your flesh for the dead, nor tattoo any marks upon you . . . " For many Jews, the idea of tattooing also brings to mind the Holocaust, since Jewish prisoners were tattooed at that time as a means for identification, a process that was known as the "ka-tzetnik identification system."[11] Islam also forbids tattooing, although new converts who had previously been tattooed are permitted to practice the faith without fear of criticism.

Still, some people, like British performing artist Marisa Carnesky, are trying to push the limitations of such established beliefs. Carnesky, who is Jewish, is heavily tattooed. She believes that by making a choice to defy Jewish law, she is "shatter[ing] the conventions of traditional theater and offer[ing] a haunting exploration of Jewish superstitions, folklore, and religious rituals and symbols."[12]

It seems that body modification is seen as acceptable in more and more circles, including those circles that connect people of faith. In 2006, Mary Fordham, features editor for the *North Greenville College Newspaper*, a publication with ties to the Southern Baptist Convention, explored the newfound acceptance of tattoos among Christian youths. While Fordham's interviews with North Greenville College faculty yielded mixed results, the students she interviewed expressed a certain comfort with their body modification choices.

"[Having tattoos] has not harmed my relationship with God, it's made it better,"[13] said John Head, a North Greenville College sophomore majoring in marketing. "If I'm feeling down, I look at my arm and see the rosary with 'God is my strength' and it's a positive motivation. [The tattoos] are a constant witnessing tool because people see them and ask what the tattoo is and why I have it. Some people who don't believe in God ask me and I'm able to explain more about God and the Bible, and I wouldn't have been able to before."[14]

David Howell, also a North Greenville College sophomore, took issue with body modification. He said, "According to scriptures, at least I know the Bible states not to make any permanent marks on your body."[15]

The fact that this discussion is happening at all shows great strides toward acceptance of body modification on the part of some conservative Christians.

If you are interested in learning more about why people get tattooed, you can do some research on your own by gathering anecdotal evidence. Anecdotal evidence is stories gathered from people with experience. If you admire someone's body modification and think you might like to try it yourself, ask that person why he or she decided to get his or her tattoo or piercing; what the process was like; or if he or she regrets the experience. Each person's answers will be unique and may or may not reflect or influence your own choices.

Chapter Four

What Does Your Body Art Reveal?

Participants with tattoos and/or body piercings were more likely to have engaged in risk-taking behaviors and at greater degrees of involvement than those without either.

Obtaining a tattoo or piercing will not only change your physical presence but also the way in which people relate to you. Despite what you may think, people will judge you either favorably or unfavorably based on your appearance. Having visible body modifications may ultimately affect your ability to get the job or internship you want, meet and impress the people you desire, and/or gain acceptance to groups including the armed services. Consider how having a tattoo or piercing might make you feel during your prom, on your wedding day, or even after becoming a parent.

FIRST IMPRESSIONS

Getting a tattoo or piercing can have an effect on your relationships with family, friends, and everyone you come in contact with for the rest of your life. You've likely heard people say, "You never get a second chance to make a first impression." There's wisdom in that statement. People consider our appearances when they first meet us and use the information they gather to help them form an opinion. As people get to know us, they form more detailed impressions of our true selves, but that first impression is an important starting point.

Your body modification sends messages to the people you meet. Different people will attach different meanings to those messages. While some people might see your piercing and think you are fashionable, hip, and adventurous, others will interpret your appearance as a statement against mainstream society. They will think that you embrace an alternative lifestyle. Others might think that your body modification is an indication that you engage in risky behaviors. Put more simply, having a body modification will get you "in" with some crowds and keep you on the fringes of others. You should consider the social implications of your body modifications before you make your decision to obtain them.

WHAT DOES YOUR TATTOO SAY ABOUT YOU?

Like it or not, there is plenty of research to suggest that people who have tattoos or piercings are more likely to use drugs and alcohol, engage in risky sexual activities, and/or strive for alternative lifestyles.

In a June 2002 issue of the *Journal of the American Academy of Pediatrics*, Sean T. Carroll, MD, a pediatrics physician at the Naval Medical Center in San Diego, California, cautioned doctors about patients who had body modifications.[1] He concluded that physicians should be aware that adolescents with tattoos and/or piercings should be questioned about risky sexual practices; offered advice about safe-sex choices; and asked about eating disorders, drug and alcohol use, and suicidal thoughts.

According to the results of Carroll's survey, "Participants with tattoos and/or body piercings were more likely to have engaged in risk-taking behaviors and at greater degrees of involvement than those without either. These included eating behavior, gateway drug use, hard drug use, sexual activity, and suicide. [A higher degree of] violence was also associated with males having tattoos and with females having body piercings."[2]

Abraham Lincoln said, "You can please some of the people some of the time, and most of the people most of the time, but you can't please all of the people all of the time." People still repeat this quote because it's very true. You can't be all things to all people, but over the course of your life, you will need to be some things to some people. It's wise to take a moment to consider how your body modification will hinder your ability to be the person you need to be in order to feel happy and accepted at different stages throughout your life and by different people.

You obviously can't plan for every moment you'll experience in the future, but you can draw upon your current life experiences to imagine some of the changes you might encounter. It is likely that you already play different roles in life. You are a son or daughter to your parents, a brother or sister to your siblings, and a grandchild to your grandparents. Perhaps you've noticed differences in the way you present yourself to your various family members. Similarly, you might present yourself differently to your friends than you do to your family. Maybe you're aware of the differences in the way you present yourself to people you've known for a long time, as opposed to people you've met more recently. Wherever you recognize the differences, you'll notice that the actions you take in order to put your best foot forward will likely change depending on the situation you encounter. That's true for all people; it's human nature. As long as you have contact with people, you will have various and changing relationships.

In School

Some school dress codes prohibit visible body modifications. If your school is one of them, you could be forced to remove your jewelry or cover your tattoo during school hours. You might even be expelled if you don't comply with school policies.

Jesse Taylor, teen author of the column "Young Blood" for modifiedmind.com, is also a peer educator. She speaks to public school groups about the pros and cons of body modification. In her column, she discusses the effect her piercing had on her public school life.

> I attended a high school that did not allow visible piercings. My septum [spike] was allowed, however, much to the chagrin of my principal, based on the wording of the student handbook.

> The piercing itself was not visible, only the jewelry . . . I see a septum spike as perfectly normal, whereas most members of my community see it as an exotic eyesore—some sort of tribal taboo—but one thing seems clear: when you cross the social barrier of acceptance and add something non-uniform, all is lost . . . [3]
>
> My principal jokingly referred to me as Brahma (a stab at the "bull ring" I wore). You can rest assured that this year's school handbook has changed the dress code a little, adding a rather vague clause that basically ruins any freedom the students had. It now states, "The District prohibits any clothing or grooming that in the principal's judgment may reasonably be expected to cause disruption of or interference with normal school operations."[4]

Today, Jesse is homeschooled to avoid the dress-code limitations that are found in most public schools across America. But if being homeschooled or dropping out of school limits your abilities to meet your personal goals, you may want to weigh the personal importance of being modified against the importance of achieving your educational ambitions. Whether it's right or wrong, having a body modification quickly becomes more than an aesthetic choice. It is important to note that school is not the only place where you might struggle with these choices. These same issues follow many adults into their professional lives, too.

In the Workplace

One of the areas in which having a body modification is most challenging is in the workplace. If you've talked to professionals about your interest in a body modification, you've possibly heard someone say, "Oh, you'll never get a job with that!" Their concern for your future career is valid. While there is evidence that body modifications are becoming more common and acceptable in a variety of situations, they are a far cry from fitting into the American standard of business casual. In many instances, your employer may ask you to cover visible tattoos and remove jewelry while you are working, which is within his or her legal rights. Employers are permitted to impose dress codes as long as they do not discriminate based on an employee's gender, race, ethnicity, religion, or age.

While concealing a tattoo or piercing might go against your personal ethics, consider the following results from the Employment Law Alliance: According to its 2005 poll, "Thirty-nine percent of Americans believe employers should have the right to deny employment to someone based on [his or her] appearance, clothing, piercings, body art, or hairstyle."[5]

Some people will tell you that their workplace easily accepts their tattoos and piercings. After years of getting body modifications, many performing artists and professional athletes are meeting less opposition to their body art. People who are employed by more casual establishments such as nightclubs, coffee shops, record stores, fitness clubs, and hair salons sometimes find their tattoos and piercings to be status quo.

For instance, Sean Cunningham, a creative director at Mullen Advertising in Weham, Massachusetts, has an arm completely covered with tattoos but does not feel that it has put a damper on his career. His opinion is quite the opposite, a fact that was revealed in a 2006 article in the *Boston Globe*.

"Usually the tattoos are an asset," said Cunningham. "Because of what I do here, people are fine with tattoos. Sometimes I actually think they feel better when they see my arm because they almost expect an artist to be tattooed."[6] Unfortunately for many in the modified masses, his experience is still an exceptional one.

In 2005, *Denver Post* journalist Tom McGhee stated, "Employment laws bar businesses from hiring based on age, gender, race, or religion. But the tattooed and pierced don't constitute a protected class."[7] In the article, McGhee told of a young man with plugs in his earlobes, a lip ring, and multiple tongue piercings who has lost job opportunities because of his piercings before finally finding a job at Tokeo Joe's, a restaurant that proudly hires the pierced. Others McGhee interviewed discussed hiding their tattoos during work hours and removing their facial piercing or replacing their jewelry with much smaller, subtler jewelry. McGhee quoted Fred Thompson, who heads up a Denver-based recruitment agency called Korn/Ferry International: "I can't see a Fortune 500 board warming up to a guy coming in with a nose ring. I still think it is fairly taboo."[8] The article also quotes a Vault.com survey of managers in which 58 percent said they'd be "less likely to hire a employee with a body modification."[9]

John A. Challenger, chief executive officer of the global outplacement firm Challenger, Gray & Christmas, Inc., offered an opposing opinion for a *USA Today* story on the subject. "Some employers are already having trouble finding skilled workers," he said, "and they are not going to let some body art get in the way of hiring the best qualified candidate. Plus, a growing number of employers recognize the benefits of diversity in all its forms and are embracing the unique attributes that make people stand out from the crowd."[10]

CHANGING TIMES

One employer that is changing its stand on hiring people with tattoos is the U.S. Army. Until recently, tattoos were permitted as long as a dress uniform could cover them. Currently, however, the Pentagon announced that it is changing its tune. Reacting to a changing youth culture and record-low recruiting totals, recruiters have begun to accept applicants with some neck and facial tattoos.

This policy is more liberal, but it is still far from "anything goes." A recent article in the *Los Angeles Times* offered the following excerpt from guidelines given recruiters by the Pentagon: "All tattoos that are on the neck that are not vulgar, profane, indecent, racist, or extremist are authorized as long as it does not extremely degrade military appearance,"[11] the guidelines read. The policy also forbids sexist tattoos, like "those that advocate a philosophy that degrades or demeans a person based on [his or her] gender."[12]

BODY MODIFICATIONS AND YOUR FAMILY

Your interest in tattoos and body piercing may or may not cause some issues between you and your parents. Just as there are a wide variety of feelings about body modifications among younger people, the reaction of parents can vary. A message board maintained by the University of California at Berkeley called Parents Network is home to ongoing discussions regarding teens who desire body modifications and the reactions and responses from their family members. One discussion about tongue piercing yields postings from parents with very different approaches regarding this choice.

One mother, Barbara, decided that she would encourage her daughter to do an abundant amount of research into the process before making the decision to permanently pierce her tongue. This research had to include information obtained from conversations with her pediatrician and her dentist. The parents made a "contract" with their daughter to go through this investigation process and then meet again in the future with the results of her research. At the same time, the parents conducted their own investigation into the process and its potential drawbacks. Barbara wrote,

> [W]e all found out a great deal of negative information about tongue piercing. Because of the time involved in doing the research and the nature of the contract, our daughter had a lot of time to feel that she could have her tongue pierced, there being a definite NO. We got an opportunity to develop our argument against it—or not! Our daughter decided against [getting her tongue pierced] on her own.[13]

Another person, Jennifer, who also posted on the UC Berkeley Parents Network, took a very different stand. She wrote,

> I would strongly advise against letting your daughter get her tongue pierced.

> Most dentists will tell you that in addition to trauma to the tongue, that metal implements in the mouth cause cracks in the back of the teeth that can lead to teeth and bone infections, some severe enough to require that sections of the jaw need replacing (which is painful and costly surgery). My father was a physician in San Francisco and had several patients with tongue piercings who experienced this very problem. Replacing the jaw is about $15,000 worth of surgery alone, not to mention recovery time and medications.[14]

Another parent recounted a story on the UC Berkeley Parents Network to explain how her son, who is now in his twenties, was grateful that he was never permitted to get a piercing when he wanted one at thirteen. Because he doesn't like them now, he was relieved that he had been advised against making the decision on his own.[15]

Maybe these people sound like your parents, or maybe they don't. Perhaps your parents have handed you the old line, "As long as you live under my roof, you'll do as I say" and have completely forbidden you from getting any type of body modification. In that case, you might have a difficult road ahead. The best thing you can do, if you really want to make a case for your choice, is to do your homework.

Learn everything you can about the body modification that sparks your interest. Are there any age restrictions to your choice, and if so, do you meet the age requirement? In other cases, would you first need your parents' permission? Think about why you want the tattoo or piercing. Have you given your decision significant thought? Can you thoroughly explain your interests to your parents? If so, sit down with them and discuss your decision rationally and calmly. Explain that you have researched the pros and cons of getting the body modification and offer examples of your newfound knowledge on the subject. Chances are, most parents will be more receptive when they learn that you have given your decision serious thought. Above all, learn about all of the risks associated with the procedures and share your findings with your parents. Together, you can both make an informed choice.

SPECIAL OCCASIONS

That big talk might not be the last one you have over your body modification. It's possible that your family will never be entirely comfortable with your choice. In that case, if you already have a visible tattoo or piercing, you might find that discussions about your choice resurface as a topic of family conversation whenever there's a special event on the horizon.

Parents might be dismayed at the sight of a tattoo peeking out from the edges of your prom dress, or perhaps they might be concerned about the first time your grandparents notice your nose ring from across the dining table. It is for these reasons and more that you should heavily consider all of your options before getting a permanent modification.

You may be asked to cover a tattoo if you are a part of a good friend's or family member's wedding party. Or you might be concerned with covering a tattoo when walking down the aisle yourself. In another instance, you might be concerned with how your new boyfriend or girlfriend will react after he or she learns you have tattoos and/or multiple piercings. Whatever the case, there are some options available to you.

If your piercing is healed, you can just remove your jewelry. If the area is still a noticeable piercing, you can probably conceal it with hypoallergenic cosmetics. Keep in mind, however, that you never want to use cosmetics for more than a few hours. Be sure to wash the area beforehand and then immediately after.

Wedding and beauty magazines are brimming over with questions and suggestions geared toward concealing tattoos and piercings. Some suggestions include choosing a gown with a lace overlay, or applying a flesh-toned bandage over the tattoo beforehand, further reducing its visibility. Other possibilities for camouflage include wearing a dress that includes a jacket, or wearing lace gloves.

Still, brides with their hearts set on a strapless or backless gown may find themselves with limited options. Some throw a wrap over their shoulders for the ceremony and then unleash their ink at the reception. Others try a host of cosmetics that promise to cover your tattoo on your special day. According to Rhonda Jackson, a Minneapolis-based makeup artist, these products offer some coverage, but they are very tricky to use and do not ultimately produce a tattoo-free look.

A family wedding isn't the only possible hurdle. In order to avoid rehashing the issue with displeased parents, grandparents, future spouses, and/or children, you might be asked to conceal your tattoo for family photographs and during reunions, special dinners, holiday celebrations, religious events, funerals, and a host of other occasions.

CHILDREN

It is possible that your children or grandchildren might not be entirely comfortable with your body modification. It may make them feel like they don't fit in, or they might be afraid that it will scare, or offend, their friends. This depends largely on the type of body modification you have and the personalities of your kids. But it's worth thinking over. Are you comfortable being the tattooed mom or the dad with stretched earlobes?

One father with sleeves of tattoos said he had considered tattooing his children's names on his arms as a sign of love and devotion to them, but his daughters (eight and ten years old) couldn't make up their minds about what they thought of their father's tattoos. Sometimes they thought the ink was cool, and other times they thought it was gross. He said that he got the ink when he was younger and hadn't really taken his future role as a father into consideration. From the tone of voice he used to discuss the matter, it's easy to imagine that he might do things differently today. In order to avoid wistful feelings of regret later in life, it's important to use the best decision-making process possible.

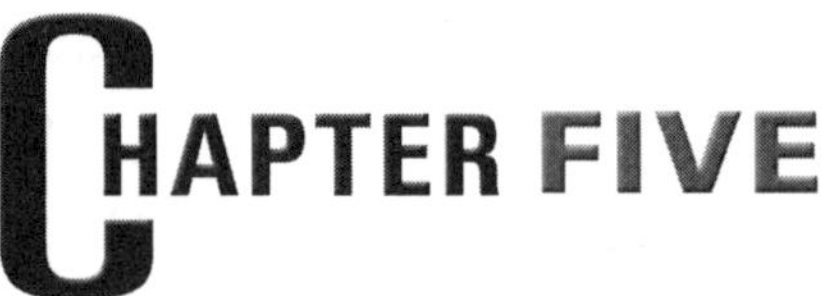

CHAPTER FIVE

Before You Make Your Decision

If a body modification sounds exciting while you're gearing up for a Goth festival, but feels less attractive when you're thinking about the prom, then you have not yet settled on your final decision.

The choice to have, or not have, a body modification is the first of many choices that you will make in your adult life. It's a great chance to try some decision-making styles and techniques to see which seem to fit your personality and lifestyle.

Most of us have some natural tendencies when it comes to making decisions. Some people make risky decisions hoping for the best possible outcome, while others avoid taking on the challenges of decision making, hoping to avoid any bad results. Some of us like to stick to safe patterns of behavior, while others jump headfirst into any challenge that catches their eye without spending much time thinking about consequences. Some people let the groups they belong to (or want to belong to) make decisions for them, while others put off making decisions altogether and accept whatever results fall their way.

None of these decision-making styles are entirely bad. There are good and bad aspects to all of them. Still, none of them are a substitute for a well-planned, carefully thought-out decision. In this chapter, we'll look at some processes that can help you make a satisfying and responsible choice about body modifications.

GAZE INTO YOUR FUTURE

Before you make any big decisions, take a moment to remember what you liked when you were ten years old. Do you remember an outfit you liked or a game you enjoyed? Maybe you remember wanting a certain toy, or had an idea of a perfect vacation spot or birthday party theme. What was your idea of a perfect Saturday morning? Quickly write down your answers to these questions.

Think about yourself today. How would you answer the same questions now? Chances are that your answers today are completely different than how you felt at ten years of age. Notice any differences or similarities in both sets of answers.

Now, if you were to ask yourself the same questions in another five or ten years, how do you think your answers would change? How about in fifteen or twenty years? The point is that people mature and their tastes change over time. People become more sophisticated and their lifestyles, responsibilities, and families change.

Keep in mind as you navigate the rest of your decision-making process that you are a growing, changing person. Spend time trying to truthfully decide if the body modification you want today will feel right to you on your wedding day, at a job interview, on a crowded beach, during a religious service, or when you meet your child's kindergarten teacher for the first time.

GATHER INFORMATION

Reading this book is a great start, but don't stop here. Read everything you can find on the topic.

Look through magazines and Web sites, and don't be afraid to gather information from the people you know who have some experience; they can be among your most valuable teachers.

TALKING IT OUT

As was previously mentioned, information gathered from friends, or from stories told by friends, is called anecdotal information. While not always the most accurate information, it can play an important part in making a healthy decision.

Begin gathering anecdotal information by making an effort to notice the people around you with body modifications. Be mindful of any reactions you have to certain modifications and styles. Some will be attractive to you, while others will not. Some styles might help you identify with the wearer, and others will make you want to steer clear of him or her. Strong reactions like these will help you narrow down your list of possible body modifications.

If you have close friends or acquaintances with body modifications, talk with them about their choices. Ask them what prompted them to have the modification. Ask about the procedure and healing process. Ask them about their friends' and family's reaction to their choice. Ask them about their own satisfaction with their decision. Listen carefully to all of the answers, but keep in mind that sometimes people, especially young people, put on a brave face in front of others. They may play down the pain they felt during the procedure or gloss over some negative reactions they may have received afterward. Given this might be the case, your friends should not be your only source of information.

ZOOMING IN

As your knowledge of body modifications grows, you may notice that your interest starts to narrow. You may find yourself very interested in a certain modification, design, color, placement, jewelry, or general style. You may start to think this is the kind of modification you'd like to have yourself. If so, you're ready to develop a focus question.

This simply means defining the question you are asking yourself. As you think of a question, keep it simple. Your question can be as basic as, "Is a tongue piercing right for me?"

If you're having trouble narrowing down your focus question, you might want to start with a group of smaller questions. Your main question could be, "Is a body modification right for me?" As you kick that question around, you might want to list the types of body modifications that catch your interest. Next to each possibility, list some advantages and disadvantages of each. Keep this list with you. Add thoughts to your list as they occur to you during the day.

After time, you might notice that one or two possibilities recur frequently or rise to the top of your list. Those winning points of interest can become your focus questions. Once you have a focus question, write it down on a piece of paper and get ready for some well-organized, effective, mature decision making.

DIGGING DEEPER

Some people like to make a list of pros (reasons for making a certain decision) and cons (reasons against making a certain decision). Often people put one list on one side of a piece of notebook paper and the other list on the other side of the page.

The list can be used in many ways. One side of the paper may have many more reasons than the other. Sometimes the reasons on one side of the paper seem much more important than on the other. The lists can line up one way, but your heart leads you strongly in another direction. The lists aren't the final say; they're just a tool to help you see what you really think and feel about a certain set of options.

It's wise to do this process over a period of time. Doing it in one sitting might just tell you what decision you would make in the moment. Sometimes putting a list away and revisiting it in a few days, weeks, or months can make the process more effective. If a body modification sounds exciting while you're gearing up for a goth festival, but feels less attractive when you're thinking about the prom or your wedding day, then you have not yet settled on your final decision. If you look at your list every day for six months and agree with your decisions every time, then you might be finished thinking it over. However, if your list looks different when you're in a different mood or in a different place in your life, then you've probably not settled on your final decision.

Eventually, you will feel yourself coming to a conclusion. As you zoom in and answer your focus question, spend some time visualizing yourself with the choice you make. Notice any emotions that visualization brings up for you. See if those emotions make you want to re-examine your answer.

Discuss your desire for a certain body modification with your parents or guardian before you take the plunge. You might even want to discuss your decision to get a tattoo or piercing with a close friend to hear his or her opinion on the subject. Making a mature decision (as well as informing your family and friends) will make the process of getting modified that much easier. This is also true since you will likely need to have a parent or another adult with you during the procedure, and this way you'll avoid major surprises later.

Finally, remember that it's not the end of the world if your parents remain opposed to your decision to get a tattoo or piercing. Today, there are many temporary options such as transfer tattoos and magnetic jewelry that can achieve the same look as permanent modifications. The next chapter discusses these alternatives in further detail and describes how you can try a variety of pain-free body art designs with little cost or risk.

CHAPTER SIX

Alternatives to Tattooing and Piercing

If you need to feel funky by Friday, but are just beginning to sift through the decision-making process, it's possible that a less permanent addition to your appearance would do the trick.

Making a decision to get a tattoo or piercing takes time, and the process can be frustrating if you want to change your look right away. If you need to feel funky by Friday, but are just beginning to sift through the decision-making process, it's possible that a less permanent addition to your appearance would do the trick. In some instances, you may even prefer the temporary nature of the following body art options.

BINDI

Maybe you've noticed the red dots some Indian women wear on their foreheads? In Hindi culture, the red dot is made from a mixture of spices and powders, like vermillion and saffron, which is applied like makeup and worn by married women. This red dot signifies their status as matriarchs and is believed to bring them good luck and prosperity.

Variations of this dot have become somewhat fashionable in Western culture. In America, wearing a bindi doesn't need to signify marriage; it can just be worn for adornment. (Although, if you're going to borrow this tradition, it's probably wise to learn a little something about it.) People who wear bindi for fashion often opt for the sticker bindi rather than applying it with paint or cosmetics. Sticker bindi are easily applied, easily removed, and available in a variety of colors, shapes, and styles. Some have crystals, sequins, and tiny beads.

Some bindi are small and meant for the face, but others are larger-sized patches meant for tattoo-like placement. They're inexpensive (many of them cost less than $20) and can be bought online or at some trendy jewelry shops.

Wearing bindi might be a great warmup—or substitute for—getting a facial piercing. Bindi are made for the forehead, the face, the eyelashes, and the fingernails. A quick browse of one of the many online shops selling bindi could easily yield several ideas.

If one catches your eye, you can experiment with alternative placements of the bindi, to see where you like having a little shimmer. Wearing them below your eyes like teardrops or on your dimples for a little extra flash might be fun. They're a no-risk way to enjoy a trend and make an individual statement. With a little creativity, you can find colors, shapes, and placements that are uniquely yours.

MEHNDI

Mehndi are long-lasting and intricate designs painted on the skin with paste made from henna leaves, which are ground into a powder and mixed with liquids such as eucalyptus oil. Mehndi (also called mehendi or mehandi) has a long history of being used in places like the Middle East, North Africa, and South Asia. Like a tattoo, mehndi can be applied to any body part, although it is traditionally found on the palm side of hands, on feet, and sometimes on the face in ornate designs. The henna paste is painted on the skin with a brush or penlike bottle. The paste dries over a period of several hours and is then peeled off, leaving an auburn-colored design on the skin. (Applying heat from a hair dryer or the sun can usually darken the color.)

While tattoos are permanent because the ink is injected deep into the skin, henna merely dyes the skin's top layers, which are naturally shed over time, making it possible for you to experience a few weeks of the mehndi without committing to a permanent design.

TEMPORARY TATTOOS

Temporary tattoos have come a long way since when they could be found on the sides of gum wrappers. Today, a range of very convincing, colorful, and fashionable designs are available in trendy shops and online.

Wet-application temporary tattoos and airbrushed tattoos are quite beautiful, painless, and possible to change as frequently as your moods allow. They can be a great quick fix for someone teetering on the edge of a snap decision or a nice addition to your cosmetics for a special party or outing, especially for those of you who are underage. Experimenting with temporary tattoos may also help you decide whether or not a real tattoo is a good choice. You might decide that a tattoo is not right for you after experiencing a similar temporary design for a few days.

HAIRSTYLE

If you're looking to make a bold statement with your appearance, you might consider a dramatic haircut or alternative hair color. If you're naturally blonde, you can simply wash in some midnight blue or cupcake pink and have a fun, attention-getting fashion accessory for the next few weeks. (Be sure to use a temporary hair color product for this option.) If you want to cultivate a more goth or punk look, black hair dye is an effective and time-honored classic. Again, be sure to try a wash-in product rather than a permanent dye.

Not only will your new hair look fantastic, it's a great way to see if you really like attracting attention from strangers with your appearance. People still turn their heads to see an unusual haircut or a flamboyant hair color. If after a week of purple bangs you wish you could just fade into the wallpaper, then maybe those stretched earlobes are for someone else. Also, you should keep in mind that many professional dress codes forbid unnatural hair colors, so a theatrical hairstyle or color could come at the cost of your after-school or summer job.

MAGNETIC JEWELRY

Those of you who are curious about nose or ear piercing might want to first try magnetic jewelry to experiment with similar looks. It's a low-cost, painless, and risk-free way to add a little extra sparkle when you feel like a change. And parents who object to an alternative piercing might be willing to discuss your desire for a nose ring after they've adjusted to your new appearance. Magnetic jewelry is also a great alternative to traditional piercing for people who are concerned about the risks from allergic reaction to certain metals such as nickel.

NON-PIERCING JEWELRY

Another low-cost, risk-free option to body piercing is to try non-piercing jewelry as a precursor or substitute for a piercing. It's an almost perfect solution for the under-sixteen set whose parents refuse to sign for a piercing. Non-piercing jewelry allows you to attach a metal ring to your eyebrow, nose, lip, or other areas. The rings stay on when gently pinched closed. They are a much lower-risk way to get the same look, and nobody will know the difference!

Many body art Web sites, like those listed in the For More Information section of this book, now carry non-piercing jewelry made to create the look of a capture ball belly ring, a pierced lip, a pierced eyebrow, or alternative ear piercing. They are often less expensive than starter jewelry for a new piercing and less likely to cause an allergic reaction. They're an accessible and legal way for younger people to enjoy an alternative look without feeling the needle.

You can experiment with just one of these suggestions or any combination of them without fearing that you have made a hasty choice or one that will later cause you grief. Have fun!

CHAPTER SEVEN

A Lifelong Commitment

IF YOU FIND YOURSELF QUESTIONING YOUR DECISION ONCE YOU'VE MADE PLANS, IT IS ABSOLUTELY OK TO CANCEL OR POSTPONE YOUR SESSION.

It's good you have such great decision-making practices under your belt because the decision to get a body modification will set off a chain reaction of other decisions that need to be made.

First, you need to decide what kind of modification you'd like. It's likely that by now you've narrowed your list of options to a few favorites. If you're thinking about a body piercing, you'll want to choose a location and type of jewelry, keeping in mind that the choices for your initial jewelry are limited by practical requirements such as gauge, construction, and metal. If you're waffling a bit on your decision, stop by piercing studios (or Web sites) and review portfolios or gallery pictures of clients. This will give you a good idea of the kind of work that an artist or studio does and will give you a sneak peek at some fresh piercings so you'll know what to expect. If, however, you're thinking of getting a tattoo, this is the time to settle on a design.

TATTOO DESIGNS

Examine a few books, articles, or Web sites written by body modification artists in which they discuss what makes a good tattoo design. If there's a tattoo parlor near you, it might be a fun idea to stop in and look at flashes (the paper drawings of tattoo designs that hang on the walls in many studios) or ask to see a portfolio. This will give you an idea of practical design styles. While at the studio, resist the urge to make an impulse decision because the design you choose will be with you for the rest of your life. You'll want to make sure that you like it, that it represents you well, and that it is meaningful to you. Getting a tattoo is not an impulsive decision.

If you're planning to have a set of tattoos or an entire sleeve done over the course of your life, this is a good time to begin thinking about a theme so that your collection of tattoos has enough commonality between them to match. (For example, some themes might include anime characters, Celtic designs, fantasy characters and fairies, or a rockabilly theme with pin-up girls and Las Vegas icons.)

ANATOMY OF A TATTOO

The artists at Texas Tattoo offer this description of the anatomy of a tattoo in the FAQs section of their Web site. "A tattoo is made up of several different components. The three major ones are the outline, the black shading, and the color. Each of these requires a different machine [setting] and technique. The outlines should be consistent in thickness and definition. The shading should be smooth and have good transition from dark to light. The color should be laid in solid without 'holidays' [breaks]. These qualities combined should result in a tattoo that will stand the test of time."[1]

A strong, well-articulated tattoo usually originates from a simple, uncluttered design. When you are considering certain designs, keep in mind the types of drawings you used to see in coloring books. Coloring book images have clear outlines, are usually limited to one or two easily recognizable icons, have limited detailing, and make clear the difference between areas to be shaded, colored, or outlined.

Once you've gotten an idea of the types of designs that work as body art, start keeping an eye out for design material in the world around you. Magazine art, stationary, graphic T-shirts, stickers, doodles by friends, and other people's body art can offer a wealth of inspiration.

If you find a design that is even close to what you want, it's wise to bring a picture of it to potential tattoo artists. This will help the artist re-create the design in the drafting stage. This is an important step! Have you ever gone to a salon for a haircut, described the style of your dreams to your stylist, and then left the salon with something completely different from what you imagined? Stylists, piercers, and tattoo artists are talented, but they are not mind readers. Having something that displays the design or style that you intend can go a long way toward bridging any communication gaps, ultimately ensuring that you get the design you want.

It's also possible that the artist you have in mind will see your design choice and refer you to another artist. This doesn't mean that he or she doesn't like you or your design. It's simply that every artist has his or her own style, talent, and ability, and some artists are a better fit for your needs. If this happens, meet with the recommended artist. You may be very glad you did.

FINDING A BODY ARTIST

Once you've located a few artists who do the kind of work you're looking for, see if you can visit their space or speak with them before setting up an appointment. It is important that you feel comfortable with the artist and the space, and that he or she is properly trained and licensed. Also, examine the studio: Is it clean? Are the restrooms clean? Has it been inspected by health officials? Look for certificates on the wall and note the inspection dates.

If you have a friend getting a tattoo or piercing, going along to his or her session will give you a great idea of whether or not this is something you'd like for yourself. Keep in mind, however, that not all parlors will let friends and/or family attend the session. In some cases, it's actually against state law for anyone else to be present.

The Alliance of Professional Tattooists' Web site offers the following advice for people choosing a tattoo artist: "Your concerns are twofold. You need to find an artist whose work you like, [and] who will work on you safely. Ask people where they got tattooed, especially if you really like the work you see. Ask to see photographs of the artist's work. Most often, the pictures will have been taken right after the work was completed, so redness and swelling are common. In spite of that, there are things you can learn. Are the lines clean and smooth, or broken and jagged? Do they meet up? Does the artist work in the style you are looking for? Taking time to check out a few artists and shops will ensure that you are happy with your results."[2]

KNOWLEDGE IS POWER

Only informed consumers can make informed choices. Before deciding on any particular tattoo artist, you should consider asking him or her the following questions.

- Is your equipment reuseable?
- Do you use an autoclave to sterilize your reuseable equipment?
- Do you use separate disposable and prepackaged sterile needles for each client?
- Do you wear disposable gloves during the procedure?
- What kind of training do you have? Is there a certificate available?
- Are you licensed by the state?
- What are the state or local requirements for inspection at this shop?
- Are your needles sterile and disposed of properly?

ASK ABOUT YOUR SESSION

Once you've found a parlor and artist that seem like a good fit for you, ask about a session. You'll want to ask about his or her pricing (keep in mind that body modification sessions can be very expensive, though some artists will negotiate their fees). It's OK to ask him or her if there's "wiggle room" in his or her pricing, but you need to be ready to accept the fact that he or she may not budge. Also, there's nothing wrong with telling the artist that you need to save up for a session, if indeed you do. Just tell him or her that you'll call when you're ready.

Just as you tip waiters and hairdressers, it's expected that you'll tip your body modification artist. The general rule is a minimum of 10 percent of the price of your modification, and 20 to 25 percent if you found the work excellent. Keep this in mind as you budget for your modification.

If you find yourself questioning your decision once you've laid plans, it is absolutely OK to cancel or postpone your session. Don't worry about what people think; it is likely that deep down they will respect you for making a decision that's right for you.

PREPARE FOR YOUR SESSION

As your appointment gets closer, reread the section of this book that discusses what to expect from your session. Refresh your mind about the risks and complications associated with the body modification you've decided upon so you can ask appropriate questions. Make sure you meet all the age, health, and other requirements of your body art studio prior to your arrival. Also, make sure you and your family are in agreement regarding permission for your modification. You want as few surprises and stressors on your session day as possible.

Finally, have a ride to and from your session. You may be too distracted to drive afterward. You might be just fine, but there's no need to risk it. Enlist a supportive and reliable friend or relative as your chauffeur for the day.

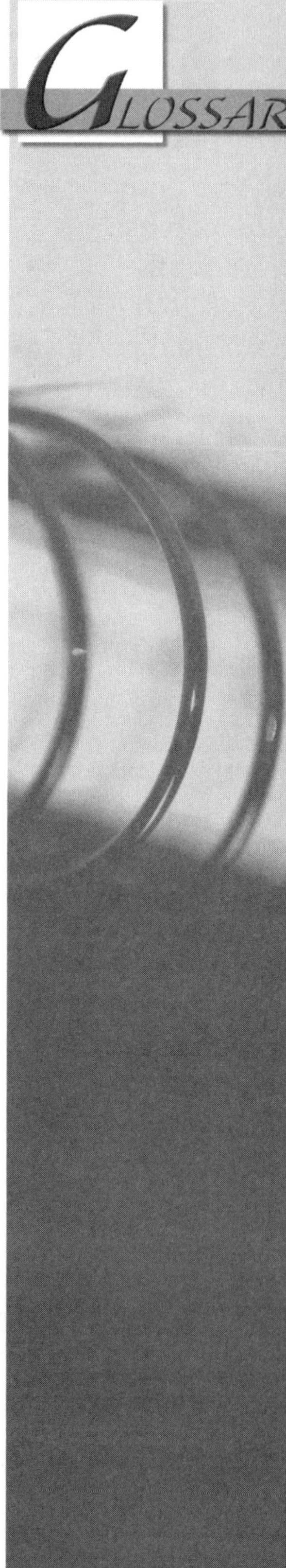

anthropologist A person who studies the origin, cultural development, and behavior of man.

autoclave A machine that uses steam at a high temperature to sterilize surgical instruments and tools.

avant-garde Of or belonging to the arts; a term often used to describe a person, especially an artist, who is ahead of his or her time.

dermatologist A doctor who specializes in the diagnosis and treatment of diseases of the skin, hair, nails, and mucous membranes.

eyelet In piercing, a style of jewelry with a large hollow center.

flash Selection of tattoo designs that hangs on walls of tattoo parlors.

fresh ink A term that describes a new tattoo, or one where the ink appears glossy.

granuloma Nodules of inflamed human tissue.

hepatitis A viral disease involving inflammation of the liver. Scientists now know there is a higher incidence of hepatitis among those people who have tattoos.

irezumi A style of ancient Japanese tattooing often using designs that cover large portions of the human body.

keloid An overgrown mass of scar tissue at the site of a healed skin injury.

labret An object that pierces the skin below the lips and above the chin.

mehndi The application of intricate temporary designs on the hands and feet with a henna paste. Mehndi originated in countries in North Africa, the Middle East, and South Asia.

moko The art of tattooing as practiced by the Maori of New Zealand and worn by men and women. Its basic and most important design element is the spiral.

rite of passage Ceremony that celebrates an important event in a person's life.

septum The part of the nose that separates the two nostrils.

tatau The Polynesian word for "tattoo."

Wicca A religion that deifies a group of natural gods, including a mother earth goddess, and that inspires worshippers by the practice of benign witchcraft.

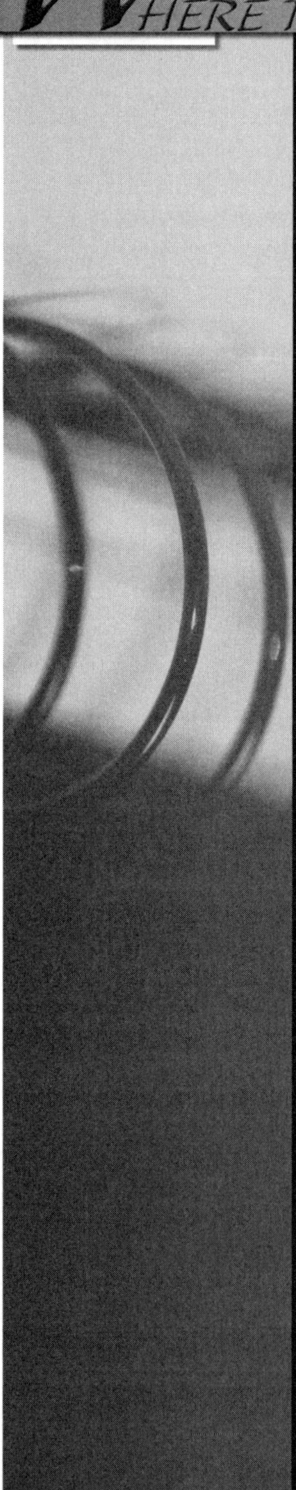

Alliance of Professional Tattooists
9210 S. Highway 17-92
Maitland, FL 32751
(407) 831-5549
Web site: http://www.safe-tattoos.com

The Alliance of Professional Tattooists is a non-profit, educational organization that was founded in 1992 to address health and safety issues facing the tattoo industry.

American Society for Dermatologic Surgery (ASDS)
5550 Meadowbrook Drive, Suite 120
Rolling Meadows, IL 60173
(847) 956-0900
Web site: http://www.asds-net.org

The American Society for Dermatologic Surgery was founded in 1970 to promote excellence in dermatologic surgery and foster the highest standards of patient care.

Association of Professional Piercers
P.O. Box 1287
Lawrence, KS 66044
(888) 888-1277
Web site:http://www.safepiercing.org

The Association of Professional Piercers is dedicated to the dissemination of health and safety information to piercers, health care providers, and the public.

Body Art Supply, Inc.
4233 SE 182nd Avenue, #169
Gresham, OR 97030
(888) 994-3662
(503) 674-2639
Web site: http://www.bodyartsupply.com

Body Art Supply, Inc., specializes in providing consumers with safe, low-cost alternatives to permanent tattooing and piercing, including temporary tattoo transfers, decals, henna, and magnetic and non-piercing earrings.

National Tattoo Association
485 Business Park Lane
Allentown, PA 18109
Web site: http://www.nationaltattooassociation.com

The National Tattoo Association was founded in 1976 to heighten awareness about tattooing as a contemporary art form. It has since become an organization dedicated to the advancement in quality, safety standards, and professionalism in the tattooing community.

WEB SITES

Due to the changing nature of Internet links, Rosen Publishing has developed an online list of Web sites related to the subject of this book. The site is updated regularly. Please use this link to access the list:

http://www.rosenlinks.com/ccw/bpta

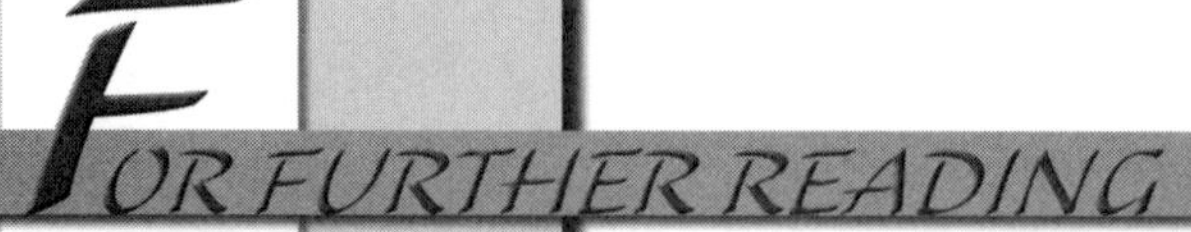

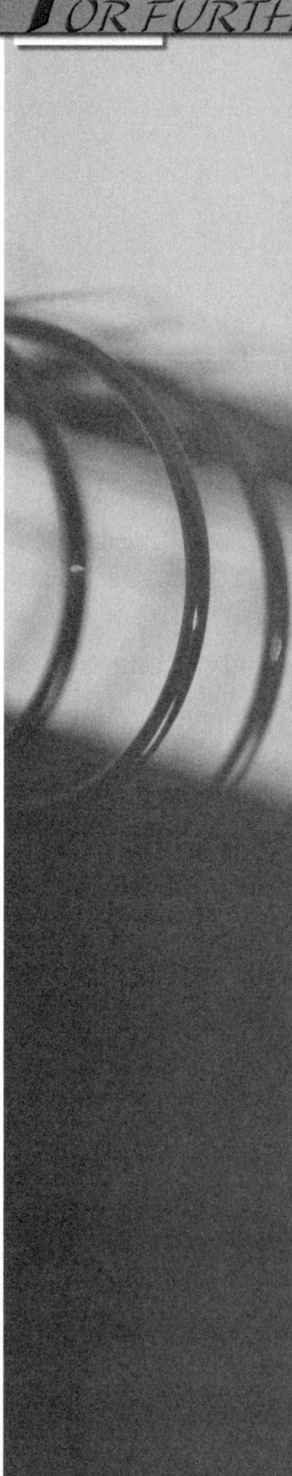

Demello, Margo. *Bodies of Inscription: A Cultural History of the Modern Tattoo Community*. Durham, NC: Duke University Press, 2000.

Gilbert, Steve. *The Tattoo History Source Book*. New York, NY: Powerhouse Books, 2004.

Green, Terisa, Ph.D. *Ink: The Not-Just-Skin-Deep Guide to Getting a Tattoo*. New York, NY: NAL Trade, 2006.

Groning, Karl. *Decorated Skin: A World Survey of Body Art*. New York, NY: Thames & Hudson, 2002.

Mason, Paul. *Need to Know Body Piercing and Tattooing* (Need to Know). Portsmouth, NH: Heinemann Library, 2004.

Mifflin, Margot. *Bodies of Subversion: A Secret History of Women and Tattoo*. New York, NY: Powerhouse Books, 2001.

Parry, Albert. *Tattoo: Secrets of a Strange Art*. Mineola, NY: Dover Publications, 2006.

Winkler, Kathleen. *Tattooing and Body Piercing: Understanding the Risks* (Teen Issues). Berkeley Heights, NJ: Enslow Publishers, 2002.

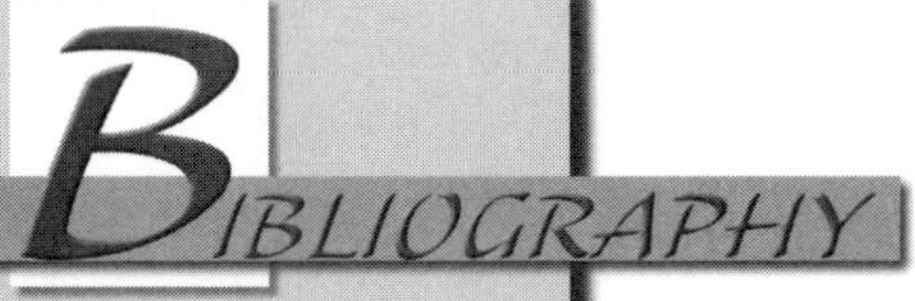

Ackerman, Diane. *The Natural History of the Senses*. New York, NY: Random House, 1991.

Barnes, Geraldine. "Curiosity, Wonder, and William Dampier's Painted Prince." *Journal for Early Modern Cultural Studies*. Retrieved July 10, 2006 (http://muse.jhu.edu/cgi-bin/access.cgi?uri=/journals/journal_for_early_modern_cultural_studies/v006/6.1barnes.pdf).

Carroll, Lynne, and Roxanne Anderson. "Body Piercing, Tattooing, Self-Esteem, and Body Investment in Adolescent Girls." *Adolescence*, Vol. 37, No. 147, Fall 2002, pp. 627–638.

Cho, David. "A Chance for a Clean Start: Tattoo Removal Programs a Tool in Anti-Gang Fight," *Washington Post*, T-3, February 20, 2005.

Cunningham, Patricia A., and Susan V. Lab. *Dress and Popular Culture*. Bowling Green, OH: Bowling Green University Press, 1991.

Dauge-Roth, Katherine. "Demon Marks Lay Bare the Twisted History of Tattooing." *Academic Spotlight*. Retrieved July 5, 2006 (http://www.bowdoin.edu/news/archives/1academicnews/ 001563.shtml).

Finan, Eileen. "Is Art Just Skin Deep?" *Time* (European edition). Retrieved July 5, 2006 (http://www.time.com/time/europe/magazine/article/0,13005,901020429-232672,00.html).

Florangela, Davila, "Redefining Beauty: Tattoos Mark Spiritual Journey of Healing from Mastectomies." Knight Ridder Tribune News Service, March 15, 2006.

Franklin-Barbajosa, Cassandra. "Tattoo: Pigments of Imagination." NationalGeographic.com. Retrieved July 5, 2006 (http://magma.nationalgeographic.com/ngm/0412/online_extra.html).

Fullard-Leo, Betty. "Body Art." *Coffee Times*. Retrieved July 5, 2006 (http://www.coffeetimes.com/tattoos.htm).

Hawthorne, Mark. "The Tale of Tattoos." *Hinduism Today*. Retrieved July 5, 2006 (http://www.hinduismtoday.com/archives/2001/7-8/38-41_tatoo.shtml).

Jesitus, John. "Body Art Risks Exposed." *Dermatology Times*. Retrieved June 20, 2006 (http://www.dermatologytimes.com/dermatologytimes/article/articleDetail.jsp?id=157808&&pageID=2).

Kreahling, Lorraine. "The Perils of Needles to the Body." *New York Times*. Retrieved July 10, 2006 (http://www.nytimes.com/2005/02/01/health/policy/01tatt.html?ex=1265000400&en=aec99feb293659bd&ei=5088&partner=rssnyt).

LaFee, Scott. "Skin Deep." *San Diego Union-Tribune*. Retrieved July 10, 2006 (http://www.signonsandiego.com/uniontrib/20060503/news_lz1c03body.html).

Mazzetti, Mark. "Army's Opposition to Ink Fading." *Los Angeles Times*, March 30, 2006, p. A-5.

McCabe, Mike. "The New York City Tattoo: The Origins of a Style." Tattoos.com. Retrieved July 5, 2006 (http://www.tattoos.com/bowery.htm).

McClain, Buzz. "Is There a Ring in Your Future?" 123DropShip.com. Retrieved July 5, 2006 (http://www123dropship.com/BodyJeweryInYourFuture.htm).

Reuters Health Staff Writers. "Superbug Outbreaks Linked to Unlicensed Tattooing." *Medline Plus*. Retrieved July 5, 2006 (http://www.nlm.nih.gov/medlineplus/news/fullstory_35402.html).

Roberti, J. W., E. A. Storch, and E. A. Bravata. "Sensation Seeking, Exposure to Psychosocial Stressors, and Body Modifications in a College Population." *Personality and Individual Differences*, Vol. 37, 2004, pp. 1,167–1,177.

Roberts, Timothy A., and Sheryl A. Ryan. "Tattooing and High-Risk Behavior in Adolescents." *Journal of the American Academy of Pediatrics*, Vol. 110, No. 7, August 2002, pp. 1,058–1,063.

Scalla, Sheen. "U.S. Debut of Marisa Carnesky's Jewess Tattooess." Science Blog. Retrieved July 10, 2006 (http://www.scienceblog.com/community/older/archives/O/a/ucl1475.shtml).

Trager, James. *The New York Chronology*. New York, NY: HarperCollins Publishers, 2003.

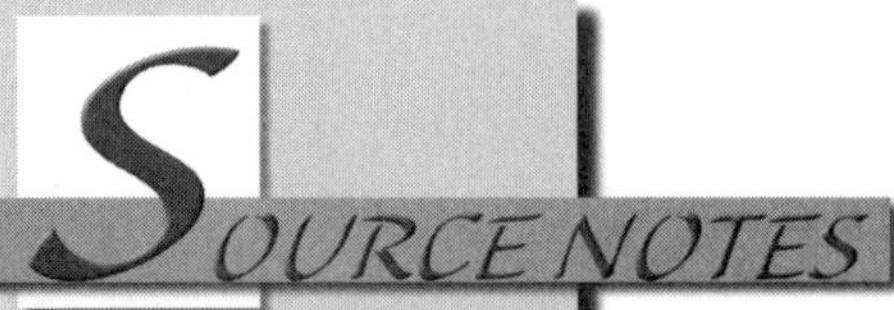

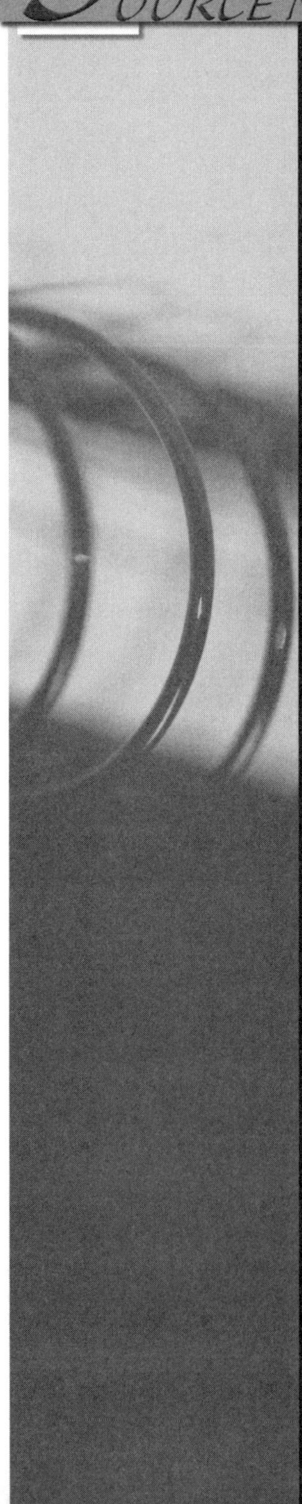

Chapter One

1. "Graffiti of the Soul," University of Massachusetts online. Retrieved July 5, 2006 (http://www.people.umass.edu/aes1/final_2.html).
2. Ibid.
3. "Bodies of Cultures: A World Tour of Body Modification," University of Pennsylvania Museum of Archaeology and Anthropology. Retrieved July 5, 2006 (http://www.museum.upenn.edu/new/exhibits/online_exhibits/body_modification/bodmodintro.shtml).
4. Karen Thomas. "States Take Stab at Regulating Teen Body Piercing," *USA Today*. Retrieved June 25, 2006 (http://pqasb.pqarchiver.com/USAToday/access/42986801.html).
5. Buzz McClain. "Is There a Ring in Your Future?" Retrieved July 5, 2006 (http://www.123dropship.com/BodyJewelryInYourFuture.htm).
6. Ibid.
7. Ibid.
8. "The Tale of Tattoos," *Hinduism Today*. Retrieved July 5, 2006

(http://www.hinduismtoday.com/archives/2001/7-8/38_tatoo.shtml).
9. Cassandra Franklin-Barbajosa, "Tattoo: Pigments of Imagination," National Geographic Online. Retrieved July 5, 2006 (http://magma.nationalgeographic.com/ngm/0412/online_extra.html).
10. Bob Cullen. "Testimony from the Iceman," Smithsonian.com. Retrieved July 5, 2006 (http://www.smithsonianmagazine.com/issues/2003/february/iceman.php?page=1).
11. "Demon Marks Lay Bare the Twisted History of Tattooing," Bowdoin College online. Retrieved July 5, 2006 (http://www.bowdoin.edu/news/archives/1academicnews/001563.shtml).
12. Ibid.
13. "Tattoo," Wikipedia.com. Retrieved July 5, 2006 (http://en.wikipedia.org/wiki/Tattoo).
14. "Body Art," *Coffee Times*. Retrieved July 5, 2006 (http://www.coffeetimes.com/tattoos.htm).
15. Ibid.
16. Ibid.
17. Ibid.
18. Diane Ackerman, *A Natural History of the Senses* (New York, NY: Random House, 1991), p. 100.
19. Ibid.
20. Geraldine Barnes, "Curiosity, Wonder, and William Dampier's Painted Prince," *Journal for Early Modern Cultural Studies*, Spring–Summer 2006, pp. 31–50.
21. Eileen Finan, "Is Art Just Skin Deep?," *Time*. Retrieved July 5, 2006 (http://www.time.com/

time/europe/magazine/article/0,13005, 901020429232672,00.html).
22. Ibid.
23. Kim Gove, et al., "Chesapeake Bay: Our History and Our Future," Mariner.org. Retrieved July 5, 2006 (http://www.mariner.org/chesapeakebay/native/nam002.html).
24. Mike McCabe, "The New York City Tattoo: The Origins of a Style," Tattoos.com. Retrieved July 5, 2006 (http://www.tattoos.com/bowery.htm).
25. Dagfinn Rognerud, "Tattoos—Techniques of Application," Ezinearticles.com. Retrieved July 5, 2006 (http://ezinearticles.com/?Tattoos---Techniques-of-Application&id=201320).
26. Cassandra Franklin-Barbajosa, "Tattoo: Pigments of Imagination."
27. Arthur Jones, "Disappearing Tattoos," Highbeam.com. Retrieved July 5, 2006. (http://www.highbeam.com/library/docFree.asp?DOCID=1G1:74439300).
28. Irving, John, "A Conversation with the Author," Randomhouse.com. Retrieved July 28, 2006. (http://www.randomhouse.com/rhpg/rc/library/display.pperl?isbn=9780345479723&view=qa).
29. Chuck Brank, "Lyle Tuttle: Forefather of Modern Tattooing," Prickmag.net. Retrieved June 20, 2006. (http://www.prickmag.net/lyletuttleinterview.html).
30. Ibid.
31. Mecca Shakoor, "The Resurgence of Body Ornamentation and Augmentation in Current

Western Civilization," Mcnair-berkeley.edu. Retrieved July 26, 2006 (http://www-mcnair.berkeley.edu/98journal/mshakoor).

32. Scott LaFee, "Skin Deep: The History and Meaning of Body Art Is Hardly Superficial," Signonsandiego.com. Retrieved July 5, 2006 (http://www.signonsandiego.com/uniontrib/20060503/news_lz1c03body.html).

Chapter Two

1. Kevin Orfield, "Tattoo Parlors Connected to Hepatitis C Epidemic," *Dermatology Insights*, Fall 2001, p. 28.
2. Ibid.
3. Reuters staff writers, "Superbug Outbreaks Linked to Unlicensed Tattooing," Medlineplus.com. Retrieved July 5, 2006 (http://www.nlm.nih.gov/medlineplus/news/fullstory_35402.html).
4. Ibid.
5. John Jesitus, "Body Art Risks Exposed," *Dermatology Times*. Retrieved June 20, 2006 (http://www.dermatologytimes.com/dermatologytimes/article/articleDetail.jsp?id=157808&&pageID=2).
6. Yannette Traver, "Body Piercing in Teenagers," byu.edu. Retrieved July 5, 2006 (http://students.cs.byu.edu/~guyatbyu/Health%20452%20Body%20Piercing.doc).
7. Ibid.

8. Lorraine Kreahling, "The Perils of Needles to the Body," *New York Times*. Retrieved July 20, 2006 (http://www.nytimes.com/2005/02/01/health/policy/01tatt.html?ex=1265000400&en=aec99feb293659bd&ei=5088&partner=rssnyt).
9. Ibid.
10. William E. Keene, Amy C. Markum, and Mansour Samadpour, "Outbreak of Pseudomonas aeruginosa Infections Caused by Commercial Piercing of Upper Ear Cartilage," *Journal of the American Medical Association*, Vol. 291, February 25, 2004, pp. 981–985.
11. Kreahling, "The Perils of Needles to the Body."
12. Ibid.
13. Ibid.

Chapter Three

1. Lynne Carroll and Roxanne Anderson, "Body Piercing, Tattooing, Self-Esteem, and Body Investment in Adolescent Girls," *Adolescence*, Vol. 37, Issue 147, Fall 2002, pp. 627–638.
2. Ibid.
3. University of Florida Study, "Piercings Are a Girl's Best Friend? Body Art Study Shows Gender Preferences," Sciencedaily.com. Retrieved July 20, 2006 (http://www.sciencedaily.com/releases/2004/12/041203084256.htm).
4. Amy Krakow, *The Total Tattoo Book* (New York, NY: Warner Books, 1994), p. 91.
5. Michael M. Phillips, "Tattoos Honor Marines Killed in Iraq and Help the Survivors," *Wall*

Street Journal. Retrieved June 20, 2006 (http://online.wsj.com/public/article/SB113996642135774155-k8VXHXAEGuXywn9QtZqXqOaDt74_20070215.html?mod=blogs).

6. Ibid.
7. David Cho, "A Chance for a Clean Start: Tattoo Removal Programs a Tool in Anti-Gang Fight," *Washington Post*. Retrieved June 20, 2006 (http://www.washingtonpost.com/wp-dyn/articles/A11232-2005Feb9.html).
8. Ibid.
9. Shawn Tussler, Interview by the author, Minneapolis, MN, June 5, 2006.
10. Davila Florangela, "Redefining Beauty: Tattoos Mark Spiritual Journey of Healing from Mastectomies," *Seattle Times*, March 15, 2006, p. 1.
11. Staff writers, "Tattoo," Economicexpert.com. Retrieved July 25, 2006 (http://www.economicexpert.com/a/Tattoo.html).
12. Scalla Sheen, "U.S. Debut of Marisa Carnesky's Jewess Tattooess," Scienceblog.com. Retrieved July 5, 2006. (http://www.scienceblog.com/community/older/archives/O/a/ucl1475.shtml).
13. Mary Fordham, "Younger Christians Okay with Tattoos," *North Greenville College Newspaper*. Retrieved June 20, 2006 (http://www.ngcskyliner.com/media/storage/paper284/news/2006/03/01/News/Younger.Christians.Okay.With.Tattoos-1641275.shtml?norewrite200608301710&sourcedomain=www.ngcskyliner.com).

14. Ibid.
15. Ibid.

Chapter Four

1. Sean T. Carroll, MD, et al. "Tattoos and Body Piercings as Indicators of Adolescent Risk-Taking Behaviors," *Journal of the American Academy of Pediatrics*, Vol. 109, No. 6, June 2002, pp. 1,021–1,027.
2. Ibid.
3. Jesse Taylor, "Young Blood," Modifiedmind.com. Retrieved June 20, 2006 (http://www.modifiedmind.com/yblood.html).
4. Ibid.
5. Staff writers, "In Many Workplaces, Tattoos Still Taboo," hr.blr.com. Retrieved July 28, 2006 (http://hr.blr.com/display.cfm/id/15210).
6. Christopher Muther, "Visible Ink," Boston.com. Retrieved July 28, 2006 (www.boston.com/yourlife/fashion/articles/2006/03/16/visible_ink?mode=PFChristopher Muther).
7. Tom McGhee, "Would You Hire This Woman?," *Denver Post*. August 14, 2005, p. A-1.
8. Ibid.
9. Ibid.
10. *USA Today* Staff Writers, "Tattoo, Bling Craze Raises Hiring Issues," *USA Today*. April 2006. Vol. 134, Iss. 2731, pg. 10.
11. Mark Mazzetti, "Army's Opposition to Ink Fading," *Los Angeles Times*. March 30, 2006. p. A-5.

12. Ibid.
13. "UCB Parents Advice About Teenagers, 'Piercings'," Parents.berkeley.edu. Retrieved June 20, 2006 (http://parents.berkeley.edu/advice/teens/piercing.html#tongue).
14. Ibid.
15. "UCB Parents Advice About Teenagers, 'Piercings'," Parents.berkeley.edu. Retrieved June 20, 2006 (http://parents.berkeley.edu/advice/teens/piercing.html).

Chapter Seven

1. Owner, Texas Tattoo Emporium, "FAQs," Texastattoo.com. Retrieved July 5, 2006 (http://www.texastattoo.com/frequently_asked_questions.htm#What%20makes%20a%20good%20tattoo).
2. Dennis Dwyer, The Alliance of Professional Tattoo Artists. "Basic Guidelines for Getting a Tattoo," Safe-tattoos.com. Retrieved July 5, 2006 (http://www.safe-tattoos.com/faq.htm).

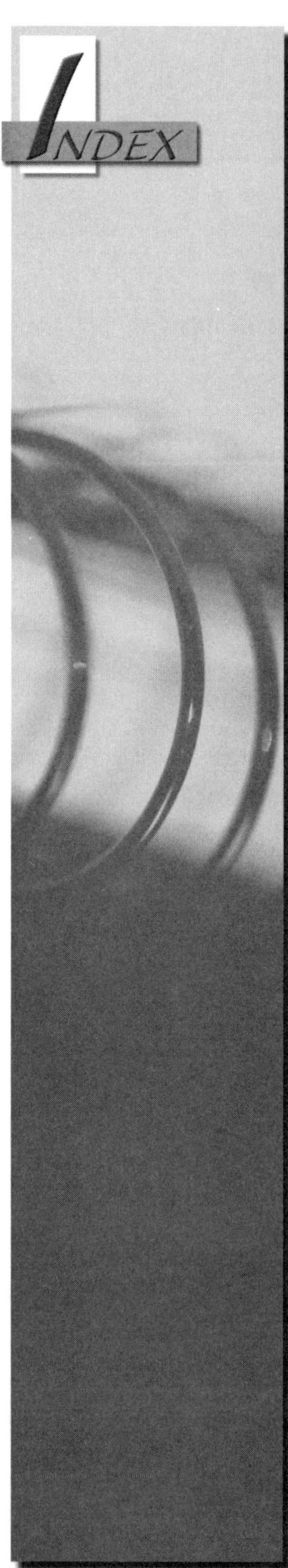

Index

A

B

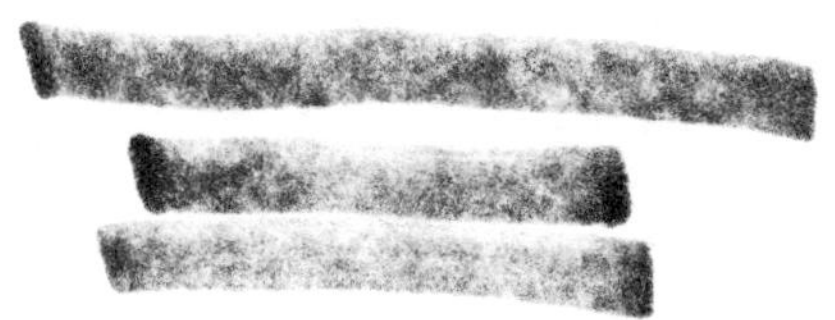

ABOUT THE AUTHOR

Sarah Sawyer has pierced ears. Her other piercings have been removed, and except for a keloid over one of them, they have healed beautifully. They were fun while they lasted. She is an arts, culture, and lifestyle writer based in Minneapolis, Minnesota.

ACKNOWLEDGMENTS

Thank you to David Sawyer, Charlotte Short, Virginia and Robert Sawyer, Marshall and Izora Devine, Daniel Sawyer, Rick Sawyer, and Bob Galloway, all of whom have provided me the years of encouragement—and the liberal arts education—it took to have the skills necessary to write this book. Thanks also to Alison Aten for her publishing guru-ness; Oliver Sewell for taking the long naps that gave me time to write; Bob's Java Hut for warm seats and hot coffee; and Joann Jovinelly for her work on this project.

Photo Credits: Cover, p. 1 © www.istockphoto.com

Designer: Nelson Sá; **Editor:** Joann Jovinelly